CULTURALLY COMPETENT COMPASSION

Bringing together the crucially important topics of cultural competence and compassion for the first time, this book explores how to practise 'culturally competent compassion' in healthcare settings – that is, understanding the suffering of others and wanting to do something about it using culturally appropriate and acceptable caring interventions.

This text first discusses the philosophical and religious roots of compassion before investigating notions of health, illness, culture and multicultural societies. Drawing this information together, it then introduces two invaluable frameworks for practice, one of cultural competence and one of culturally competent compassion, and applies them to care scenarios. Papadopoulos goes on to discuss: how nurses in different countries understand and provide compassion in practice; how students learn about compassion; how leaders can create and champion compassionate working environments; and how we can, and whether we should, measure compassion.

Culturally Competent Compassion is essential reading for healthcare students and its combination of theoretical content and practice application provides a relevant and interesting learning experience. The innovative model for practice presented here will also be of interest to researchers exploring cultural competence and compassion in healthcare.

Irena Papadopoulos is Professor of Transcultural Health & Nursing at Middlesex University, UK.

CULTURALLY COMPETENT COMPASSION

A Guide for Healthcare Students and Practitioners

Irena Papadopoulos

DATE DUE

Routledge
Taylor & Francis Group

LONDON AND NEW YORK

CONTENTS

All chapters have been written by Irena Papadopoulos except Chapters 2 and 3,
which have been co-authored with Sue Shea.

FOREWORD

By Julia Puebla Fortier

DIRECTOR, DIVERSITYRX – RESOURCES FOR CROSS CULTURAL HEALTH CARE

We live in a world of rapidly changing demographics and a disorientating range of claims about the benefits and challenges of increasing mobility. On the one hand, societies are enriched by the hardworking, entrepreneurial drive of immigrants and the vibrant social and cultural diversity they bring to the communities where they set down roots. On the other hand, differentness can raise anxiety about social and economic insecurities propelled by the larger forces of globalisation.

Responding to and fanning these anxieties, politicians and pundits try to shape social narratives to promote agendas of retreat from our interconnectedness. Stained by xenophobia, name-calling and cynicism, our ideals of a progressively more tolerant society are under threat. But in the clinic, the hospital ward and the community, healthcare providers must keep their minds focused on the business of care and caring. It is all too easy to let the toxic narratives unconsciously impact the way we see and interact with others who may be different from us – socially, culturally, educationally, economically.

The rationale for cultural competence in healthcare has evolved over the decades, from human rights and social justice to patient safety and reducing inequalities. Elaborated through a multiplicity of model programmes, policies, training initiatives and research, it has found legitimacy in the agendas of health systems, national governments and international organisations. Alongside the calls for more patient-centred care, cultural competence has informed an understanding that patients are more than biological bodies that require expert 'fixes' – they have unique personal characteristics that shape how they receive and respond to the interpersonal act of healing.

The heart of healthcare is care itself – attending to the needs of individuals in a time of need or crisis. Care and healing compels an act of vulnerability on the part of both the carer and those receiving care. For the carer, this requires developing and nurturing an inner capacity for empathy and concern that is enacted as compassion. Sadly, all too often in the practice of modern medicine, the imperative is something else – efficiency, cost savings, technology. These forces often override the time and space that all healthcare providers need to engage in the act of compassionate care.

This textbook invites us to engage in a self-reflective process that involves learning about others, but also learning about ourselves – the origins of our values and the deeper examination that is possible when we engage in a dialogue with the frameworks of many traditions. It takes us on a thought-provoking journey through the philosophical and religious underpinnings of compassion and elucidates the concepts and practices related to compassionate care and culturally competent care, then joins the two together. In so doing, we see that one cannot be considered without the other and that the two concepts enrich each other and offer a paradigm to fully understand and empathetically interact with those in our care. It is this combination of the concepts and tools of both cultural competence and compassionate care that offers us a way to shape our actions and reactions when confronted with situations outside our personal experiences.

As the book moves from the philosophical to the practical, the reader sees that the insights and approaches presented are grounded in years of research, practice, teaching and dialogue with those engaged in culturally competent and/or compassionate care. The many phases of the Intercultural Education of Nurses in Europe initiative have yielded a wealth of material that has been transformed into clear and sensible concepts designed to inform, guide and engage the reader. Each chapter ends with questions that consolidate and personalise learning by prompting a self-examination of current attitudes and future behaviours.

The book highlights the interpersonal nature of developing attitudes and behaviours that are culturally compassionate. Some learning can be acquired in books, but we imitate what we see. So role models in teaching and in leadership are essential to shaping and supporting good practice. At the same time, Papadopoulos makes the case for an empirical examination of culturally competent compassion. While the concept may invoke an intangible, inner quality, the associated actions can be assessed and measured, and there are many opportunities and challenges for improving our ability to do so.

We must not overlook the reality that the good intentions and actions of individuals need to be supported by organisational norms and structures that support compassionate care. Truly attentive and empathetic interactions require time. Nurses and other healthcare staff are often squeezed by impossible demands and high expectations. It is hard to give when you are distracted and depleted. Those who are involved in planning, implementing and financing health services would be well-served to incorporate the concepts of culturally compassionate care into their decision-making.

The book ends with a surprising leap into the future – the world of culturally competent compassionate robots. While technological interventions may seem the antithesis of human care, it is both brave and forward-thinking to confront the inexorable move to incorporating care services provided by 'thinking machines'. Can compassion be programmed? Can harmful stereotyping or bias be eliminated? Papadopoulos is on the cutting edge of addressing these questions, and the whole scope of this important textbook will prepare learners at all levels to take culturally competent compassion into this radical transformation of healthcare.

ACKNOWLEDGEMENTS

I wish to thank all those colleagues and students who, over the years, contributed to my personal, professional and academic development journeys in their own unique ways. Permit me to mention some of my most recent co-travellers: Alfonso Pezzella, Laura Foley, Akile Zorba, Sheila Ali, Sue Shea and Christina Koulouglioti. I thank them for their support during the preparation of this book.

I want to acknowledge the cooperation I received over the last ten years from my European partners of the Intercultural Education for Nurses (and other health professionals) in Europe (IENE) projects (1–6), especially Victor Dudau.

I am also grateful to my many international collaborators for their enthusiastic contributions to our international culturally competent compassion efforts.

My final big thank you goes to my family, especially my husband, Costas, whose support continues to be unwavering and uniquely compassionate.

1

INTRODUCTION

My 25-year journey of discovering cultural competence and compassion

Introduction

I spent the first 20 years of my academic life conducting research aimed at illuminating the notion of cultural competence in healthcare practice. I have tackled research questions such as:

*   Why do we need to take culture into consideration when learning to care?
*   What is cultural competence?
*   Why should healthcare-providing institutions be culturally competent?
*   How and what should be included in the healthcare curricula in order to promote cultural competence?

In my quest to answer these and other questions, I reviewed the literature and nursing curricula, I observed teachers in classrooms and practitioners in clinical areas, I conducted numerous interviews and I attended international conferences. Eventually, this culminated in the creation and further elaboration of the Papadopoulos, Tilki and Taylor (1998/2006) model for the development of culturally competent practitioners. I was, however, aware that whilst some research-evidenced content was being developed – particularly by nurse researchers in the USA – specific content addressing the UK cultural and structural issues was lacking. My response was to design and lead a number of studies that explored the health and care needs of minority ethnic groups, refugees, asylum seekers and Gypsy Travellers. These studies explored the importance of cultural identity, cultural values, the impact of culture on the understanding of health and illness and self-care practices, the barriers encountered when attempting to access healthcare services and the broader socio-cultural determinants of health.

I had defined cultural competence as "the process one goes through in order to continuously develop and refine one's capacity to provide effective health care, taking into consideration people's cultural beliefs, behaviours and needs" (Papadopoulos, 2006, p.11). Since all human beings are cultural beings, it is clear that culturally competent care is the most desirable approach to healthcare for all people. Further, I had always believed that culturally competent care was compassionate care! However, in 2010, my first and second grandchildren were born. Due to pregnancy complications of one of my daughters-in-law, I spent some time accompanying her to her hospital appointments prior to and after the delivery of the baby. It was at this time that I realised that many midwives (including student midwives) were not only culturally incompetent, but also they appeared indifferent to the suffering of my daughter-in-law and son. Upon reflection on all my observations, I concluded that the midwives I had met lacked compassion.

In February 2010, Sir Robert Francis QC published his first report into the shocking scandal of negligence at the Stafford hospital. The report was the stimulus for an unprecedented discussion on compassion by the mass and social media. Many professional and academic journals began to feature articles on compassion, with many authors asserting that, in some hospitals, dignity, care and compassion are routinely absent. The Department of Health together with the NHS Commissioning Board published in 2012 their three-year strategy 'Compassion in Practice Nursing, Midwifery and Care Staff. Our Vision and Strategy' stating that:

> The compassion and humanity we show shapes the culture of our health service and our care and support system. We care for everyone, from the joy at the beginning of new life to the sadness at its end. …We support the people in our care and their families when they are at their most vulnerable and when clinical expertise, care and compassion matter most. But there are big challenges. People also encounter care that falls short of what they have a right to expect, sometimes by a long way. We know we miss too many opportunities to support people to keep well, connected and healthy. …We must seize this opportunity to create a future where people are placed at the heart of care and are treated with compassion, dignity and respect by skilled staff who have the competence and time to care, a future where the unbounded potential of our professions to provide compassionate care, promote independence, health and well-being is properly unleashed…

The strategy was underpinned by the following values: care, compassion, competence, communication, courage and commitment (www.england.nhs.uk/wp-content/uploads/2012/12/compassion-in-practice.pdf).

Amongst all the efforts to address the lack of compassion, numerous solutions, strategies and analyses of the related issues were offered, none of which acknowledged the fact that in the twenty-first century UK (and indeed in most countries), which has multicultural service users and multicultural service providers, compassion, whilst being a universal value, nevertheless has culture-specific meanings and ways of enactment.

What you will find in this book

This book deals with 'culturally competent compassion', which I have defined as a

> …human quality of understanding the suffering of others and wanting to do something about it using culturally appropriate and acceptable caring interventions which take into consideration both the patients' and the carers' cultural backgrounds as well as the context in which care is given.
>
> *(Papadopoulos, 2011)*

It is therefore clear to see that this book brings together the notions of cultural competence and compassion in a unique synthesis relevant to practice.

This book constitutes essential reading for undergraduate healthcare students, who will find the combination of theoretical content and practice application a relevant and interesting way to learn. It is proposed that the recent alarming reports about the care void of compassion strongly indicate a need for all healthcare workers to consider the essence of care, which is culturally competent compassion. This book will provide the tools for such consideration.

Before one attempts to learn how to practice culturally competent compassion, it is important to have a strong foundation about its theoretical building blocks. This process begins with Chapters 2 and 3, which discuss the philosophical and religious roots of compassion. You will find that there is an Aristotelian connection in the topics discussed and the propositions made in this book. Other important building blocks are the notions of health, illness, culture and multicultural societies and the Papadopoulos, Tilki and Taylor model of cultural competence (1998/2006), all of which will be addressed in Chapter 4. Chapter 5 discusses the meaning of compassion and why this is essential to nursing. The constructs of the Papadopoulos model for culturally competent compassion will be explored and applied to care scenarios. The views and challenges of learning to be a compassionate care provider are discussed in Chapter 6, which will also examine how students are taught and supervised during their practice placements. Chapter 7 continues with this theme, but focuses on the role of leaders at different levels of the organisation and their responsibility of being compassionate role models, supporters of those in their charge and creators of compassionate working environments. Chapter 8 examines the issues relating to researching compassion and reports on the findings of an international survey of compassion that I conducted in 2014–2015 with a group of talented volunteer researchers from 15 countries. This survey endeavoured to identify how nurses in different countries defined and provided compassion to patients and to highlight their views on whether compassion is being taught in nursing courses, whether they believed patients valued compassion over technical competence and whether they (the nurses) received compassion and by whom. The last topic to be addressed in Chapter 9 is the controversial issue of whether we could or should be measuring compassion – ideally, of course, the culturally competent compassion type. The book ends with Chapter 10, which presents some of my reflections regarding the future of culturally competent compassion.

References

Commissioning Board Chief Nursing Officer and DH Chief Nursing Adviser (2012). *Compassion in Practice*. Retrieved from www.england.nhs.uk/wp-content/uploads/2012/12/compassion-in-practice.pdf.

Papadopoulos, I., Tilki, M. and Taylor, G. (1998). *Transcultural care. A guide for health care professionals*. Dinton, UK: Quay Publications.

Papadopoulos, I., ed. (2006). *Transcultural health and social care: Development of culturally competent practitioners*. Edinburgh, UK: Churchill Livingstone Elsevier.

Papadopoulos, I. (2011). Courage, Compassion and Cultural Competence. Paper presented at the *13th Anna Reynvaan Lecture*. De Stadsschouwburg – Amsterdam City Theatre, the Netherlands.

Francis, R., The Mid Staffordshire NHS Foundation Trust Inquiry (2010). *The independent inquiry into care provided by Mid Staffordshire NHS Foundation Trust January 2005–March 2009*. London, UK: The Stationary Office.

2

PHILOSOPHICAL ROOTS OF COMPASSION

By Irena Papadopoulos and Sue Shea

LEARNING OBJECTIVES

Upon completion of this chapter, readers should be able to:

- Demonstrate a basic knowledge of the views and arguments put forward by the six philosophers outlined in this chapter and how these relate to compassion.
- Demonstrate a basic understanding of how historical viewpoints can be applied to ethical and moral aspects of modern-day clinical practice.
- Recognise the importance of applying the work of philosophers to our current understanding of the various aspects of compassion such as self-compassion, compassion fatigue and compassionate leadership.
- Describe the differences and similarities between the six philosophers' explanations of compassion.
- Reflect on what you have read and relate it to your own practice.

Introduction

The term 'philosophy', meaning 'love of wisdom', represents an activity that people undertake when they seek to understand fundamental truths about themselves, their relationships with each other, the world in which they live and their relationships with the world. Scholars of philosophy are consistently engaged in asking, answering and arguing for their answers to life's most basic questions (https://philosophy.fsu.edu/undergraduate-study/why-philosophy/What-is-Philosophy).

Philosophy and healthcare do not exist in isolation. Whilst what constitutes healthcare may be complex, what constitutes philosophy can also be complicated, as both may introduce moral dilemmas. Furthermore, both contain aspects of the relationship between mind and body.

Knowledge of historical viewpoints with regard to compassion can be helpful in our understanding of how the concept is utilised and understood in modern-day healthcare settings. Furthermore, the study of philosophy can help us to understand the different components to compassion, such as self-compassion and compassionate leadership (see Chapters 5 and 7).

Although it is generally thought that Greek and Roman philosophers distrusted the concept of compassion, believing that reason alone was the proper guide to conduct, compassion has been deliberated by scholars since Aristotle's days (van der Cingel, 2014). Compassion and related terms appear in the early writings of Aristotle and Confucius and represent central concepts in both early and contemporary Buddhism (Goetz, Keltner and Simon-Thomas, 2010).

This chapter seeks to briefly explore perspectives of compassion from six key philosophers: Confucius, Aristotle, Hume, Schopenhauer, Nietzsche and Gandhi. We have tried to point out how their thinking converges and where it differs. It is important to note that the chosen philosophers lived in different parts of the world and in different times, both of which impacted on the cultures of the societies our philosophers grew up in or lived in and undoubtedly these cultures would have also impacted on their thinking. Philosophy as exemplified by the philosophers dealt with in this chapter addresses the question of how we should live and how we should approach and understand our fellow human beings.

Confucius – 551–479 BCE – Chinese teacher, editor, politician and philosopher

> Wisdom, compassion and courage are the three universally recognised qualities of men.
>
> *(Attributed to Confucius)*

Confucius was an influential Chinese philosopher who is known for his models of social interaction. His teachings focused on creating ethical models of family and public interaction and setting educational standards. According to Chinese tradition, Confucius was a thinker whose teachings formed the foundation of much of the subsequent Chinese speculation relating to the education of the ideal man, how individuals should live their lives and interact with others and the forms of society within which they should participate (http://plato.stanford.edu/entries/confucius/).

Confucius emphasised that people should have compassion towards each other and should not treat others in ways that they themselves would not wish to be treated. In order to be compassionate, people should avoid self-aggrandisement and practice altruism and self-restraint (http://confucius-1.com/teachings/). His philosophy emphasised personal morality, justice, sincerity and correct social relationships.

Confucius taught that the heart and mind defines the uniqueness of being human, and thus he insisted on empathising and extending virtues to others as a method of cultivating humanity (Ng, 2009). He is believed to have authored many classic Chinese texts, including all of the Five Classics. His teachings were collected in the *Analects*, which were compiled by his disciples and by his followers many years after his death. Within the *Analects*, compassion is expressed in Confucius' call to leaders to exemplify a moral nobility and to act with kindness, loyalty and faithfulness (Opdebeeck and Habisch, 2011; http://plato.stanford.edu/entries/confucius/).

Confucius' principles were based on common Chinese traditions and beliefs. He believed in strong family loyalty, ancestor worship and respect of elders by their children. Furthermore, he recommended the family as a basis for ideal government (Khan and Osborne, 2005). It was believed that family members act as a social unit and obligations among members have priority over duties to those outside of the family. However, while close family members are given priority, Confucianism extends such obligations to members of the extended family and the society at large (Lee, 2015). Philosophical Confucianism encourages people to focus on family love and its societal expansion, whilst at the same time exploring humane love, mental tranquillity, care, suffering and empathy (Munro, 2016).

It would appear that Confucius' social philosophy was based on the principle of 'loving others' while exercising his own self-discipline. There is a belief that benevolence, or 'ren', constituted the Confucian path leading to the formulation of the Golden Rule – *do not do to others what you would not like them to do to you* (Low, 2011). For Confucianism, empathetic feelings are at the heart of *ren* and rest at the root of morality, requiring us to relieve the suffering of others (Lee, 2015). It was believed that *ren* could be put into action using the Golden Rule and that the concept represented the outward expression of Confucian ideals, which was seen as a Confucian virtue symbolising the good feelings that a virtuous human experiences when taking an altruistic approach towards others. *Ren* is also defined in terms of virtues such as respectfulness, loving kindness, tolerance and trustworthiness (Low, 2011). *Ren* is concerned with the belief that the greatest value in life is selfless dedication. For Confucius, benevolence is the most important character of human beings that resides in the nature of every person. Living as a caring, compassionate person, the benevolent person is passionate and enthusiastic about being benevolent (Low, 2011).

Confucius' political beliefs were further based on the concept of self-discipline. He believed that a leader needed to demonstrate self-discipline and provide a positive example in order to remain humble and treat his followers with compassion. Confucius' theory is rich in ethical thoughts about health. His theories on morality and ethics served as the 'key notes' of the traditional medical ethics of China (Guo, 1995). Followers of Confucius believed that medicine was the ultimate expression of saving people via love.

Benevolence – the core value of Confucianism – extends from the importance of familial ties and blood connections and is held in high esteem by the Chinese (Lihua, 2013). Benevolence was also concerned with respect for patients. Care was the duty of the physician and the ultimate expression of humanity, and self-cultivation was practised by Confucian physicians through self-examination, self-criticism and self-restriction (Carter, n.d.).

The viewpoints of Confucianism, including benevolence and kind-heartedness, were inherited by medical workers and as such became prominent in Chinese traditional medical ethics. This system has been followed and amended by medical professionals of all generations throughout Chinese history. It contains concepts such as the need to attach great importance to the value of life, to do one's best to rescue the dying and to heal the wounded, to show concern to those who suffer from diseases, to practice medicine with honesty, to comfort oneself in a dignified manner, to respect local customs, to treat patients equally and to respect the academic achievements of others (Guo, 1995).

The guiding principle in Confucius' social teachings is that people should love one another and treat each other with kindness, a concept that is shared by all major religions and humanistic philosophies (http://confucius-1.com/teachings/).

SUMMARY

- Confucius focused on how individuals should live their lives and interact with others.
- He believed in strong family loyalty and the family as the basis for ideal government. He placed much emphasis on benevolence as the most important characteristic of human beings.
- Many of his teachings were compiled in the *Analects* by his disciples and followers.
- Confucius' philosophy was based on 'ren' (loving others) and he was the founder of the Golden Rule (*do not do to others what you would not like them to do to you*).
- He believed that a good leader needed to exercise self-discipline in order to treat his followers with compassion.
- Confucius' theories were rich in ethical thoughts about health.
- The viewpoints of Confucianism, including benevolence and kind-heartedness, were all inherited by medical workers and as such became prominent in Chinese traditional medical ethics.
- The guiding principle in Confucius' social teachings is that people should love one another and treat each other with kindness.

Aristotle (384–322 BCE) – Greek philosopher

Although compassion is thought to involve an active moral demand to address others' suffering, it is believed that ancient philosophers such as Plato and Aristotle rejected compassion as the basis of our moral obligations because of the danger of becoming overwhelmed with emotions and because they believed in justice as the basis of moral virtue. Moral obligations in this perspective should be directed from above through tight political control. Thus, compassion and pity were viewed as the loss of moral autonomy and of self-control (Sznaider, 1998).

However, although rejecting compassion as the basis of moral obligation, Aristotle does give pride of place to compassion as an emotional virtue, describing it as the experience of pain at another person's undeserved bad fortune (Kristjánsson, 2014).

In feeling compassion, we may consider that, in the main, a good portion of another's predicament was caused in a way for which the person is not to blame. Thus, Aristotle held that compassion for the hero of a tragedy represents the viewer's belief that the hero is not responsible for his downfall (Nussbaum, 2008).

Aristotle's theory of tragedy offers a classical framework with which to think about the problems provoked by the representation of human suffering (Giraldo, 2013).

According to Aristotle in *Poetics*, a tragedy is "a classical framework with which to think about the problems provoked by the representation form; with incidents arising pity and fear, wherewith to accomplish its catharsis of such emotions" (https://ia600204.us.archive.org/5/items/thepoeticsofaris01974gut/poetc10.txt).

Tragedy, within a Greek sense, looks mainly at the relationship between man in his life and his death. For the Greeks, this meant to plot the relationships between changeable man and the unchangeable relationships between the immortal gods.

Giraldo (2013) reports that Aristotle conceived of the individual's reaction to tragedy as a combination of fear and compassion directed towards the pain of another being. Thus, for there to be compassion, we need to acknowledge a situation as something harmful for the other and that we react with pain to that harm, recognising at the same time that although this person is different from us, our shared frailty becomes a common bond. Aristotle further claims that these emotions may be provoked by the spectacle or the 'suffering' (i.e. by the physical presence of destruction on the stage), but that ideally these emotions should derive from the structure of the story itself: "For the story must have been put together in such a way that, even without seeing, he who hears the events as they come to be, shudders and pities from what occurs" (Aristotle, 2001, 1453b 1–7 in Giraldo, 2013).

Saunders (2015) argues that Aristotle's use of the word 'pity' is clearly a reference to 'compassion' as outlined in the Aristotelian definition of pity as a feeling of pain at an apparent evil that is destructive or painful, that befalls one who does not deserve it and that we might expect to befall ourselves or some friend of ours. Goetz, Keltner and Simon-Thomas (2010) report that the term 'pity' is sometimes used to describe a state close to what we conceptualise as compassion; however, pity involves the additional appraisal of feeling concern for someone considered inferior to the self.

Aristotle prioritised appraisals of deservingness, rooted in assumptions regarding the sufferer's character and intentions. He argued that those who deserved to suffer should be blamed and reproached, whilst undeserved suffering should elicit a compassionate response, suggesting that appraisals of blame are important as to whether or not compassion arises (Goetz, Keltner and Simon-Thomas, 2010). Furthermore, Aristotle defined compassion as an emotion directed at others' suffering and indicated three necessary factors: perceiving others' suffering seriously; believing this suffering is not deserved; and believing that any one of us could suffer from the same event (Taner, n.d.).

As reported by Walsh (2015), Aristotle's best human life is attained through theoretical contemplation and, similarly to Confucius, Aristotle sees the best contemplation as presupposing full ethical commitment to community life (Walsh, 2015). Thus, Walsh (2015) argues that in Aristotle's view, the best human contemplation requires one to be fully morally good, and this requires commitment to the good of others and the community. According to Scott (1995), even a brief consideration of the nature of nursing indicates that an ethical dimension underlies much or all of nursing practice. Thus, Aristotelian theories may provide a practice-based focus for healthcare ethics for a number of reasons, including the Aristotelian emphasis on the importance of perception and emotion in moral decision-making (Scott, 1995).

In an article aiming to introduce the wider philosophy of Aristotle to nurses and healthcare practitioners, Allmark (2017) suggests that Aristotle's system can be set out as a hierarchy, with metaphysics at the top and methodology running throughout. This author concludes that the goals of nursing, which are based on health, are subsumed by the overall human goal of flourishing, and this helps us to understand and set boundaries in healthcare (Allmark, 2017).

Drawing on examples from medicine in which treatment changes according to the needs of each patient, Aristotle believed that in ethics, and in life in general, mathematical exactness cannot be applied. Aristotle had a great respect for medicine, and his consideration that each person should be taken as a special case bears similarities to today's emphasis on person-centred medicine (Ierodiakonou, 2014).

Aristotle identified the primary antecedent of compassion as others' serious suffering, including specific events such as death and experiences of bodily assault or ill treatment, old age, illness, lack of food, lack of friends, physical weakness, disfigurement and immobility (Goetz, Keltner and Simon-Thomas, 2010). The application of Aristotle's work can be seen in medicine, science, ethics and other major fields of importance.

SUMMARY

- Aristotle described compassion as an emotional virtue, defining it as pain at another person's undeserved bad fortune.
- Aristotle drew on Greek tragedy to describe compassion for the hero who is not responsible for his downfall.
- Aristotle conceived the individual's reaction to tragedy as a combination of fear and compassion directed towards the pain of another being.
- He recognised that what befalls one person could befall any of us.
- Aristotle perceived compassion as being worthy of feeling towards those who are undeserving of suffering.
- Aristotle, like Confucius, saw the best contemplation as presupposing full ethical commitment to community life.
- His consideration that each person should be taken as a special case bears similarities to today's emphasis on person-centred medicine.

David Hume (1711–1776) – Scottish philosopher, historian, economist and essayist

> No [com]passion of another discovers itself immediately to the mind. We are only sensible of its causes or effects. From *these* we infer the passion: And consequently *these* give rise to our sympathy.
>
> *(David Hume, 1928, original emphasis)*

According to Himmelfarb (2008), 'benevolence', 'compassion', 'sympathy', 'fellow-feeling' and a 'natural affection for others' were the basis of the social ethic that informed British philosophical discourse for the whole of the eighteenth century. Thus, these themes were included in many of the philosophical discussions of this time.

David Hume is considered one of the first Western philosophers to emphasise compassion as the basis of morality and one of the classic proponents of moral sentimentalism (Pollock, 2014; Fotaki, 2015). According to this school of thought, our understanding of virtue arises primarily from our capacity for feeling as opposed to reason (Pollock, 2014). Hume discusses compassion or pity from the viewpoint that it represents a 'desire of happiness' and 'aversion to misery' for another person. In his opinion, these statements form the root of benevolence, and since benevolence is related to love by nature, compassion therefore is related to love. In addition to its similarity to benevolence, Hume also describes compassion as a concern for the misery of others that can be explained through sympathy. We can sympathise with others because we recognise their 'pains and pleasures'. The tragic circumstances of others evoke compassion and this requires imagination. Thus, compassion may arise from imagination, in that the realisation that certain circumstances can happen to ourselves as well as to others helps us imagine how this would be for someone else. Furthermore, Hume describes compassion as 'a kind of grief or sorrow' and as an 'uneasiness' or pain for the misery of others. As such, Hume formulates a direct link between compassion and suffering, in that to see or imagine the suffering of another person produces a form of similar suffering in ourselves (van der Cingel, 2015).

There are three statements that Hume endorses:

(1) Sympathy with those in distress is sufficient to produce compassion toward their plight;
(2) Adopting the moral point of view often requires us to sympathise with the pain and suffering of distant strangers; but
(3) Our care and concern is limited to those in our close circle.

On this basis, Hume suggests two distinct types of sympathy: we feel compassion towards those we perceive to be in distress because associative sympathy leads us to mirror their emotions, but our ability to enter into the afflictions of distant strangers involves cognitive sympathy and requires us only to reflect on how we would feel if experiencing a similar situation (Collier, 2010). Thus, in the case of distant strangers, we enter into a thought process that enables us to imagine what it would be like to experience what they are experiencing.

In *A treatise of human nature*, Vol. 2, Hume (1928) states that pity can be explained from reasoning concerning sympathy. All humans are related to each other by resemblance (presumably by our physical appearance or our physiological make-up), thus their interests, passions, pains and pleasures may affect us and produce an emotion similar to the original one. Hume argues that if this is true, it must be more so of affliction and sorrow, as these always have a stronger and more lasting influence than pleasure or enjoyment. Hume (1928, pp. 86–88) writes that

> …the spectator of a tragedy on stage (and also in real life) passes through a long train of grief, terror, indignation, and other affections which the poet represents in the person he introduces. As many tragedies end happily and no excellent one can be composed without some reverses of fortune, the spectator must sympathise with all of these changes, and receive the fictitious joy as well as every other passion.

Hume concludes that "A contrast of any kind never fails to affect the imagination, especially when presented by the subject; and it is on the imagination that pity entirely depends."

Thus, Hume maintains that our compassionate responses to those in distress are easy to explain in terms of sympathy and that we have a natural tendency to mirror the emotional states of others. We care about their welfare because we are able to feel their pain.

As such, we can apply Hume's theory to healthcare in the consideration of identifying with the suffering patient, mirroring their pain and identifying their needs.

SUMMARY

- Hume discussed compassion or pity from the viewpoint that it represents a 'desire of happiness' and 'aversion to misery' for another person.
- Hume also described compassion as a concern for the misery of others, which is to be explained through sympathy.
- He believed that the tragic circumstances of others evoke compassion and this requires imagination.
- Furthermore, to see or imagine the suffering of another person produces a form of similar suffering in ourselves.
- In explaining his theories, Hume drew upon the concept of the spectator of a tragedy on stage.
- Similarly to Aristotle, Hume placed importance on the realisation that what happens to another person could also happen to ourselves.
- Hume believed that we feel compassion towards those we perceive to be in distress because associative sympathy leads us to mirror their emotions.

Arthur Schopenhauer (1788–1860) – German philosopher

Arthur Schopenhauer had an interest in Greek tragedy and is believed to have been gripped by the misery of life, with an ultimate goal of finding a solution to suffering. He believed that humans were motivated by their own basic desires (the will to live), which directed all of humankind.

Like Hume, Schopenhauer also refers to the use of the imagination and identification with suffering. Schopenhauer refers to the mental picture of another and the identification with him/her, which leads to participation in the suffering of another, ultimately resulting in sympathetic assistance in an attempt to relieve such suffering (Schopenhauer, n.d.). Schopenhauer argued that rather than rational rules or God-given commandments, it is compassion, or *Mitleid*, that forms the true basis of morality. He believed that moral behaviour consists of an intuitive recognition that we are all manifestations of the will to live. We are united by the realisation that life itself consists of endless suffering due to the pursuit of goals that can never be satisfied. This pursuit ultimately results in a meaningless death (Madigan, 2000). Schopenhauer's compassion emphasises that a person should participate immediately in another's suffering (Downes, 2017). For Schopenhauer, a mature person is not the one who follows duty, but the one who has developed his virtues of compassion to perfection (Kakkori and Huttunen, 2016).

Schopenhauer (1972, p.43) argues that work, worry, toil and trouble are indeed the "lot of almost all men their whole life long." He refers to the imagination of an ideal world or 'Utopia' where "everything grows of its own accord, and turkeys fly around ready roasted, where lovers find one another without any delay and keep one another without any difficulty." But he concludes that in such a world, men would die of boredom, and fight and kill, thus creating for themselves more suffering than nature already inflicts on them.

Schopenhauer stated that although it would be better not to live at all, since we are alive, then we at least have a moral obligation not to *increase* suffering. We must be patient and tolerant and show charity towards other fellow suffering beings.

Schopenhauer argued that *Mitleid* as a desire for another's well-being is possible only if another's misery becomes directly the same sort of incentive as one's own misery. Thus, just as experiences contrary to one's will are painful and move one in ways to relieve such pain, in having *Mitleid* towards another's misery, the other's pain assumes the same status as one's own. As such, in individuals disposed to *Mitleid*, the apprehension of another's suffering involves "the immediate participation, independent of all ulterior considerations, primarily in the suffering of another, and thus in the prevention or elimination of it" (quoted in Cartwright, n.d.). It would appear that Schopenhauer's concept of *Mitleid* corresponds to our notion of compassion, in that it is an emotion that is directed towards another's suffering, providing an incentive to pursue the other's well-being by relieving this suffering (Cartwright, n.d.).

Schopenhauer's ethical theory was that instead of suggesting how we should behave, we should answer the question, "What moves individuals to perform actions of a particular moral value?" He claimed that by answering this question he had uncovered the 'foundations of morality'. According to Schopenhauer, actions have one of three moral values: they are either morally indifferent, morally reprehensible or possess moral worth. Schopenhauer argued that all human actions are intentional and directed to something that is either in agreement with their will or contrary to their will. He concluded that *Mitleid* is the motive for morally worthwhile actions, whilst egoism is the motive for morally indifferent actions and malice for morally reprehensible actions. As such, he viewed compassion as the motive for morally valuable actions (Cartwright, n.d.).

Thus, we may relate the work of Schopenhauer to issues with regard to our moral obligation to decrease suffering within the healthcare setting.

SUMMARY

- Schopenhauer had an interest in Greek tragedy and is believed to have been gripped by the misery of life.
- He postulated that humans are motivated by their own basic desires (the will to live).
- Like Hume, Schopenhauer also referred to the use of the imagination and identification with suffering.
- He believed that compassion is the imaginative identification of oneself with the sufferings of others.
- Rather than religion, Schopenhauer viewed compassion as the true basis of morality and the motive for morally valuable actions, the foundations of which are based on the will to live.
- Schopenhauer portrayed a rather pessimistic view of the world, stating it would be better not to live at all, but since we are alive, then we have a moral obligation not to *increase* suffering.

Friedrich Wilhelm Nietzsche (1844–1990) – German philosopher, cultural critic and poet

Like Schopenhauer, Friedrich Nietzsche admired the ways in which the Ancient Greeks used the concept of tragedy. He gave new life to the modern reception of tragedy, and for him it became a powerful label that could be applied to cultures, mentalities and historical moments (Porter, 2005).

In contrast to Aristotle, Hume and Schopenhauer, Nietzsche is believed to have been a harsh critic of compassion, and many of his publications try to expose its true motives. While he initially referred positively to Schopenhauer, Nietzsche is believed to have felt the need to draw away from his doctrine of compassion (Madigan, 2000). Thus, once a great admirer of Schopenhauer's ethics of compassion, Nietzsche later began to despise compassionate feelings (Wilkes, 2000).

Nietzsche came to see compassion as a weakness rather than a virtue, which led him to break away from what he took to be Schopenhauer's unhealthy denial of life (Madigan, 2000). Nietzsche claimed that pity is demeaning both to the pitier and to the pitied because it falsely assumes that life should be easy (Stocker, 2002). He felt that to show pity for others was to treat them with contempt, believing that it is better to encourage them to face up to their difficulties and deal with them as best they can (Madigan, 2000).

According to Nietzsche, pity increases the amount of suffering in the world by allowing us to suffer with those for whom we feel pity. Thus, our strength and will to power are minimised, simply making life more miserable (Denneson, 1999).

Like Schopenhauer, Nietzsche felt that there was a will to life underlying all existence, but he preferred to refer to this as the 'will to power'. He rejected the Enlightenment deliberations on civilisation, reason and universality, believing instead that it should be seen as a destructive creativity based on the will to power and the desire to act, stating that all formulations of moral conduct are attempts by the weak to curb the power of the strong. For Nietzsche, compassion and love represent expressions of resentment, bitterness and hatred of the lower classes of society with regard to their superiors (Sznaider, 1998).

Nietzsche believed that unless we have other options, we may purposely seek out those who are suffering to "present ourselves as the more powerful and as a helper, if we are certain of applause, if we want to feel how fortunate we are in contrast, or hope that the sight will relieve our boredom" (Cartwright, n.d., p.562).

Nietzsche claimed that compassion can be thought of in terms of power and that pity is a sentiment for the weak, suggesting that those who possess great power harden themselves against compassion. On those who possess little or no power, he says: "Pity is the most agreeable feeling among those who have little pride and prospects of great conquests: for them easy prey – and that is what all who suffer are – is enchanting" (Nietzsche, 1974, p.87).

Initially, Nietzsche understood the saint as embodying the supreme achievement of a self-transcending 'feeling of oneness and identity with all living things', but later he came to view the saint as representative of an unhealthy, life-denying 'ascetic ideal' (McPherson, 2016). According to McPherson (2016), this shift, may have been partly due to Nietzsche's development of an 'ethic of power' as part of his turn against Schopenhauer's ethic of compassion.

In Nietzsche's view, Christianity in particular was a religion of pity, basing itself upon the image of a bleeding and suffering deity (Madigan, 2000).

In Nietzsche's critique of Christianity, compassion is not rejected, but he claims that within a Christian context, compassion is driven by feelings of hatred and resentment and applied in an unhealthy way. Thus, this may be interpreted as Nietzsche believing that compassion in Christianity is as much about personal power and control as it is about selfless devotion to others: "I regarded the inexorable progress of the morality of compassion, which afflicted even the philosophers with its illness, as the most sinister symptom of the sinister development of our European culture" (Nietzsche, 2008, p.101).

According to Cartwright (n.d.), it is possible to conclude that Schopenhauer is best understood as claiming that compassion is the basis of actions possessing moral worth and that Nietzsche is concerned with showing the undesirable dimensions of pity. Thus, Schopenhauer describes an emotion that serves as an incentive that has as its end another's well-being, whilst Nietzsche discusses an emotion that has as its end the interests of the agent.

It is possible that Nietzsche's beliefs reflected his own personal experience and suffering. It is reported that Nietzsche had overwhelming personal experiences of compassion due to illness and death in his family and with his first aid activities in military hospitals during the German–French war in 1870. As a result, Nietzsche suffered from feelings of passivity and helplessness, which gave him the impression that compassion was a negative emotion (Wilkes, 2000). It is therefore possible that Nietzsche could have become overwhelmed and afraid of the concept of compassion and may have experienced an extreme level of what we today refer to as 'compassion fatigue'.

SUMMARY

- Like Schopenhauer, Friedrich Nietzsche admired the ways in which the Ancient Greeks used the concept of tragedy.
- Although he initially referred to Schopenhauer as 'the only serious moralist', he felt the need to draw away from his doctrine of compassion.
- Nietzsche came to see compassion as a weakness, not a virtue to be cultivated.
- He felt that there was a will to life underlying all existence, which he preferred to call the 'will to power'.
- For Nietzsche, compassion and love are but expressions of resentment, bitterness and hatred of the lower classes of society towards their superiors.
- Believing in the will to power rather than the will to live, Nietzsche viewed compassion as a negative emotion, stating that suffering was necessary for achievement.
- Nietzsche believed that pity is demeaning both to the pitier and to the pitied. To show pity for others is to treat them with contempt; it is not a selfless act, but rather the pitier is subconsciously thinking of himself.
- It is possible that Nietzsche's beliefs reflected his own personal experience and suffering.

Mohandas Karamchand Gandhi 1869–1948 – Pre-eminent leader of the Indian independence movement in British-ruled India

Mahatma Gandhi is noted as the benevolent leader who led India's struggle for freedom (Low, Ang and Robertson, 2012). He focused his efforts on formulating and practicing non-violent methods to end British colonialism, repeatedly warning people that he was a political activist rather than a scholar (Gier, 2015). Gandhi was born into a Hindu merchant caste family in Western India and studied law in London. After his return to India in 1915, Gandhi set about organising peasants, farmers and urban labourers to protest against excessive land taxes and discrimination. In 1921, he took over leadership of the Indian National Congress and led nationwide campaigns for easing poverty, expanding women's rights, building religious and ethnic harmony, ending untouchability and achieving self-rule (http://purehistory.org/mahatma-gandhi/).

Gandhi apparently taught that the best way to find yourself is to lose yourself in the service of others (Carr, 2016). Gandhi believed that from childhood onwards we become and stay healthy only in response to the authentic enactment of empathy by those in authority over us and the authenticity of their words and deeds rather than their words or slogans alone. He believed that this applied to any form of organised leadership and advised that we should "be the change that we wish to see in the world" (Gandhi, 1913, p.241).

Gandhi utilised the term 'non-violence' to refer to our natural state of compassion when violence has subsided from the heart. Non-violence, or 'lack of desire to harm or kill', represents the personal practice of being harmless to the self and others under every condition. It emerges from the belief that hurting people, animals or the environment is unnecessary to achieve a goal and refers to a general philosophy of abstention from violence based on moral, religious or spiritual principles (Singh and Erbe, 2017) When Gandhi wrote to a Burmese friend in 1919, he stated that when he became acquainted with the teachings of the Buddha, his eyes were opened to the limitless possibilities of non-violence (Gier, 1999). Mahatma Gandhi is regarded as a leader who brought about social change by applying his belief in non-violence and love of humanity in order to accomplish his specific goal of securing India's independence from British colonialism (Cha, 2013).

For Gandhi, the word 'non-violence' meant much more than the absence of war or the absence of violence. He believed that the practice of non-violence was concerned with people's attitudes, behaviours and relationships with each other as well as with nature and the earth. Gandhi maintained that only positive thoughts could lead to a positive destiny. He defined positive thoughts as love, respect, understanding, compassion and other positive emotions and actions. He believed that from childhood we are taught to be successful in life by any means and that such success is always measured in terms of material possessions. We therefore succumb to our egos, which leads us to extreme selfishness. As such, Gandhi set himself very high standards in his practice of ethical leadership (Dhar, 2014).

Similar to the way in which Socrates (470–399 BCE) engaged in a critical analysis of attitudes and beliefs in ancient Athens, Gandhi also presented his beliefs to the public and encouraged discussion. He understood the development of psychological and emotional self-discipline to be indispensable to the success of his socio-cultural endeavours. Gandhi felt that if he could not overcome his own impulses and unhealthy desires, he would not be able to inspire rational self-constraint and active compassion in others. Thus, Gandhi sought a simple life of rational self-governance, compassion, generosity and resilience in the face of long-term challenges (Ferraiolo, 2013).

Gandhi believed that a leader who is to serve others must be humble and that a life of service must be one of humility – the quality of being modest and respectful. Humility is widely seen as a virtue in many religious and philosophical traditions, being connected with notions of the utmost unity with the universe or the divine and living without ego. Thus, Gandhi persistently embraced and practised the value of humility (Low, Ang and Robertson, 2012).

SUMMARY

- Mahatma Gandhi is noted as the benevolent leader who led India's struggle for freedom.
- He led nationwide campaigns for easing poverty, expanding women's rights, building religious and ethnic harmony, ending untouchability and achieving self-rule.
- Gandhi believed that from childhood onwards we become and stay healthy only in response to the authentic enactment of empathy by those in authority over us.
- The term 'non-violence' as utilised by Gandhi refers to our natural state of compassion when violence has subsided from the heart.
- Gandhi is regarded as a leader who brought about social change by applying his belief in non-violence and love of humanity to accomplish the specific goal of securing India's independence from British colonialism.
- Gandhi believed that if he could not master his own impulses and unhealthy desires, he would not be able to inspire rational self-constraint and active compassion in others.
- Gandhi maintained that only positive thoughts could lead to a positive destiny, and he set himself very high standards in his practice of ethical leadership.

Concluding remarks

This chapter has identified the thoughts of six philosophers with regard to the concept of compassion. We can trace certain similarities in their views with regard to compassion and how we might apply this within healthcare settings. For example, Aristotle and Hume both recognised that events that affect another individual could also affect ourselves. Likewise, Hume and Schopenhauer refer to the use of the imagination in terms of relating to the suffering an individual's circumstances by imagining what it would be like to experience what they are experiencing. By contrast, the work of Nietzsche introduces certain complexities in terms of his harsh rejection of the concept of compassion. However, it is important to consider such an alternative view in an attempt to understand why Nietzsche differs so much in his perspective of the benefits (or lack of benefits) of compassion. It seems that four of the philosophers covered within this chapter (Aristotle, Hume, Schopenhauer and Nietzsche) all had an interest in Greek tragedy and utilised this within their work, whilst in the case of Gandhi we may perceive him as being a 'victim' of tragedy following his assassination in 1948.

Within this chapter, we have looked at philosophers' views on compassion throughout different time periods and we have covered two philosophers with Eastern backgrounds

(Confucius and Gandhi) and four with Western origins (Aristotle, Hume, Schopenhauer and Nietzsche).

Again, we can identify various similarities – despite large differences in time period – between our two philosophers of Eastern origin (Confucius and Gandhi) in that both emphasise leadership and self-discipline.

In terms of a compassionate approach within modern-day healthcare, we may argue that all of the philosophers covered provide us with profound insights and could be seen as relevant to different aspects of the concept of compassion, such as self-compassion (e.g. mirroring, imagination, self-discipline and understanding ourselves), compassionate leadership (leading by positive example) and potentially compassion fatigue (in the case of Nietzsche, who perhaps withdrew from the concept of compassion due to over-exposure to human or self-suffering).

As stated at the beginning of this chapter, a knowledge of historical viewpoints with regard to compassion can be helpful in our understanding of how the concept is utilised and understood in modern-day healthcare settings. As such, the study of philosophy can assist us in our understanding of the different branches of compassion, such as self-compassion and compassionate leadership.

To conclude, nurses face numerous dilemmas as part of their work, and making the correct and most compassionate decisions may be difficult. How do nurses decide whether their actions are always correct and beneficial or whether they may cause harm? In complex clinical environments where uncertainty is often high, how do healthcare professionals respond to the demands they face, ensuring their actions are fair and compassionate to everyone in their care? How do they know how much compassion is needed in any situation? Can an understanding of philosophy assist nurses and other healthcare workers in their choice of action? Examples of dilemmas may range from crucial decisions made during end-of-life care to more simple decisions regarding everyday procedures, as in the example that follows.

EXAMPLE A

Nurse A is on night duty at a busy London hospital. It is 3.30 a.m. and most of the patients are sleeping. One patient (Patient A), however, remains alert and is in discomfort. Patient A is awaiting surgery and has had nothing to eat or drink for several hours – she is very hungry and extremely thirsty and cannot sleep due to her anxieties concerning the forthcoming surgery.

Nurse A is concerned about the well-being of Patient A. Nurse A has received information that an accident has recently taken place and that the people involved have been taken for immediate surgery due to the injuries that they have sustained. As a result, Nurse A concludes that there is likely to be a significant delay before Patient A is taken for surgery. Although Nurse A has been instructed not to offer Patient A any food or drink, she considers that under the circumstances it would probably be safe to do so.

With the above in mind, Nurse A approaches Patient A and very quietly tells her of the current situation. Relaying the information that Patient A's surgery might be substantially delayed, Nurse A asks if she would like a cup of tea and a sandwich. Patient A immediately responds that she most certainly would. Patient A is much relieved when Nurse A brings her the tea and sandwich, and she considers Nurse A's actions to be very compassionate.

> Sometime later, the surgical team arrives to tell Patient A that they are now ready to take her for surgery. They ask the patient if she has had any food or drink prior to this moment. Wishing to avoid any trouble that this might cause to Nurse A, Patient A replies that she has not. Back in the office, Nurse A explains what she had done and proposes that enough time has already passed since the ingestion of a small sandwich to be safe for the patient to have her surgery, with which the surgical team agrees.

As with the approach of certain philosophers outlined within this chapter, Nurse A, as an observer, has knowledge of the recent tragedy that has taken place (in terms of the accident). She also has experience of how such tragedies can affect other patients (i.e. Patient A in terms of long delays). Using her discretion, Nurse A has made a decision based on similar ideas to those outlined by our philosophers in terms of imagining and identifying with Patient A's situation, sympathising with her and taking action to relieve her discomfort.

LEARNING ACTIVITIES

- Write a few notes to compare and contrast two of the philosophers' explanations of compassion discussed within this chapter.
- Write some notes on how you believe that historical viewpoints can be incorporated into everyday practice.
- Create a diagram to show how the work of philosophers may be applied to or be relevant to modern-day terms such as 'self-compassion', 'compassion fatigue' and 'compassionate leadership'.
- Think of a time when you or a colleague might have encountered a moral/ethical dilemma within the workplace – how might a knowledge of philosophy help in your understanding/actions in terms of providing culturally competent and compassionate care?

References

Allmark, P. (2017). Aristotle for nursing. *Nursing Philosophy*, 18(3), p.e12141.

Aristotle (n.d.) The Project Gutenberg E-text of *The Poetics*. Retrieved June 2017 from: https://ia600204.us.archive.org/5/items/thepoeticsofaris01974gut/poetc10.txt.

Carr, D.B. (2016). "Care" without compassion – The eighth social sin? *Pain Medicine*, 17(12), pp. 2153–2154.

Carter, B.B. (n.d.). Medical ethics – East and West. Retrieved June 2016 from: http://pulsemed.org/medethics.htm.

Cartwright, D.E. (n.d.). Schopenhauer's compassion and Nietzsche's pity. Retrieved May 2016 from: www.schopenhauer.philosophie.uni-mainz.de/Aufsaetze_Jahrbuch/69_1988/Cartwright.pdf.

Cha, M.J. (2013). Ethical values and social change: Mahatma Gandhi, Martin Luther King, Jr. and Ahn Chang Ho. *Korean Social Science Journal*, 40(2), pp. 101–111.

Collier, M. (2010). Hume's theory of moral imagination. *History of Philosophy Quarterly*, 27(3), pp. 255–273.

Confucius. (n.d.) Retrieved April 2016 from: http://plato.stanford.edu/entries/confucius/.

Confucius (n.d.). Teachings of Confucius. Retrieved June 2016 from: http://confucius-1.com/teachings/.

Denneson, T.J. (1999). Nietzsche's *The Antichrist*. Retrieved June 2017 from: https://infidels.org/library/modern/travis_denneson/antichrist.html.

Dhar, S.S. (2014). Gandhi's philosophical thoughts and debates. *Samajbodh*, 4(1/2), pp. 55–66.

Downes, P. (2017) Reconceptualising Schopenhauer's Compassion through Diametric and Concentric Spatial Structures of Relation. *Enrahonar. An International Journal of Theoretical and Practical Reason*, 58, pp. 81–98.

Ferraiolo, W. (2013). Gandhi and stoicism. *The Classical Review*, 63(2), pp. 603–605.

Fotaki, M. (2015). Why and how is compassion necessary to provide good quality healthcare? *International Journal of Health and Policy Management*, 4(4), pp. 199–201.

Gandhi, M.K. (1913). *Collected works*. New Delhi, India: Publications Division, Ministry of Information and Broadcasting, Government of India, Vol.13, Ch.153, p.241.

Gandhi, M.K. (n.d.). Pure History. Retrieved January 2017 from: http://purehistory.org/mahatma-gandhi/.

Gier, N.F. (1999). Gandhi and Mahyna Buddhism: A humanism of nonviolence and compassion. Retrieved June 2016 from: www.webpages.uidaho.edu/ngier/gbnd.pdf.

Gier, N. (2015). Gandhi, Mohandas K. *The International Encyclopedia of Ethics*, 1–8.

Giraldo, D.J.T. (2013). On art, compassion, and memory. *Proceedings of the European Society for Aesthetics*, 5, pp. 498–513.

Goetz, J.L., Keltner, D. and Simon-Thomas, E. (2010). Compassion: An evolutionary analysis and empirical review. *Psychological Bulletin*, 136(3), pp. 351–374.

Guo, Z. (1995). Chinese Confucian culture and the medical ethical tradition. *Journal of Medical Ethics*, 21(4), pp. 239–246.

Himmelfarb, G. (2008). The roads to modernity: The British, French, and American enlightenments. Retrieved October 2016 from: http://catdir.loc.gov/catdir/samples/random052/2003060576.html.

Hume, D. (1928). *A treatise of human nature*, Vol.2. Edinburgh, UK, Oxford Clarendon Press, pp. 86–88.

Ierodiakonou. C. (2014). Medicine as a model for Aristotle's ethics and his person-centered approach. *International Journal of Person Centred Care*, 4(1), pp. 31–34.

Kakkori, L. and Huttunen, R. (2016). Schopenhauer and Nietzsche on moral growth. Retrieved April 2017 from: https://link.springer.com/referenceworkentry/10.1007/978-981-287-532-7_366-1.

Kahn, K. and Osborne, K. (2005). *World history: Societies of the past*. Winnipeg, Canada, Portage and Main Press, p.117.

Kristjánsson, K. (2014). There is something about Aristotle: The pros and cons of Aristotelianism in contemporary moral education. *Journal of Philosophy of Education*, 48(1), pp. 48–68.

Lee, C.H. (2015). Intimacy and family consent: A Confucian ideal. *Journal of Medical Philosophy*, 40(4), pp. 418–436.

Lihua, Z. (2013). China's traditional cultural values and national identity. Retrieved June 2016 from: http://carnegietsinghua.org/publications/?fa=53613.

Low, K.C.P. (2011). Confucius, the value of benevolence and what's in it for Humanity? *Conflict Resolution & Negotiation Journal*, 1, pp. 32–43.

Low, K.C.P., Ang, S.L. and Robertson, R.W. (2012). Gandhi and his value of humility. *Leadership and Organizational Management Journal*, 3, pp. 105–116.

Madigan, T.J. (2000). Nietzsche & Schopenhauer on compassion. Retrieved May 2016 from: https://philosophynow.org/issues/29/Nietzsche_and_Schopenhauer_On_Compassion.

McPherson, D. (2016). Nietzsche, cosmodicy, and the saintly ideal. *Philosophy*, 91(1), pp. 39–67.

Munro, D.J. (2016). Investigation of things. *Dao*, 15(3), pp. 321–339.

Nietzsche, F.W. (2008). *On the genealogy of morals*. Oxford, UK: Oxford University Press, *p.*101.

Nietzche, F. (1974). *The gay science*. New York, NY, Random House, p.87.

Ng, R.M.-C. (2009). College and character: What did Confucius teach us about the importance of integrating ethics, character, learning, and education? *Journal of College and Character*, 10, p.4.

Nussbaum, M.C. (2008). Compassion: Human and animal. Special Lecture, delivered at the Institute of Development Studies Kolkata.

Opdebeeck, H. and Habisch, A. (2011). Compassion: Chinese and Western perspectives on practical wisdom in management. *Journal of Management Development*, 30(7/8), pp. 778–788.

Pollock, R.C. (2014). The party of humankind: Sociality and moral revision in David Hume. Retrieved April 2017 from: https://etda.libraries.psu.edu/catalog/24784.

Porter. J.I. (2005). Nietzsche and tragedy. In: R. Bushnell, ed. *A companion to tragedy*. Chichester, UK: Blackwell Publishing, p.68.

Saunders, J. (2015). Compassion. *Clinical Medicine*, 1(2), pp. 121–124.

Schopenhauer, A. (1972). *Essays and aphorisms*. Aylesbury, UK: Hazell Watson and Viney Ltd, p.43.

Schopenhauer, A. (n.d.) On the basis of morality. Retrieved April 2017 from: www.monsalvat.no/mitleid.htm.

Scott, A. (1995). Aristotle, nursing and health care ethics. *Nursing Ethics*, 2(4), pp. 279–285.

Singh, S. and Erbe, N.D. (2017). *Creating a sustainable vision of nonviolence in schools and society*. Hershey, PA: IGI Global.

Stocker, S.S. (2002). Facing disability with resources from Aristotle and Nietzsche. *Medicine, Health Care, and Philosophy*, 5(2), pp. 137–146.

Sznaider, N. (1998). The sociology of compassion: A study in the sociology of morals. *Cultural Values*, 2(1), pp. 117–139.

Taner, B. (n.d.). The role of resonant leadership in organizations. Retrieved April 2016 from: www.eujournal.org/index.php/esj/article/viewFile/1292/1301.

van der Cingel, M. (2014). Compassion: The missing link in quality of care. *Nurse Education Today*, 34(9), pp. 1253–1257.

van der Cingel, M. (2015). Why compassion still needs Hume today. *Diametros*, 44, pp. 140–152.

Walsh, S.D. (2015). Contemplation and the moral life in Confucius and Aristotle. *Dao*, 14, p.13.

Wilkes, J. (2000). The psychology of compassion. An analysis of the 100th anniversary of the death of Fredrich Nietzsche. *Psychotherapie, Psychosomatik Medizinische Psychologie*, 50(6), pp. 255–258.

3

COMPASSION AND RELIGIOUS EXPLANATIONS

By Irena Papadopoulos and Sue Shea

LEARNING OBJECTIVES

Upon completion of this chapter, readers should be able to:

- Demonstrate a basic knowledge of the values, beliefs and practices of the five religions outlined in the chapter and how these impact on compassion.
- Demonstrate a basic understanding of the relationships between religion, culture and compassion.
- Have a deeper understanding of their own personal values and beliefs.
- Recognise ways in which their own religiosity, spirituality and beliefs might affect how they provide care to patients.
- Understand the implications of religious practices and beliefs on compassion in healthcare.
- Demonstrate an awareness that religiosity, spirituality and cultural beliefs are important elements of the health and well-being of patients.
- Describe the differences and similarities of the five religions in terms of their explanations of compassion.

Introduction

The first wording to be utilised in relation to 'compassion' is thought to date back to 500 BCE when Confucius formulated the Golden Rule *do not do to others what you would not like them to do to you*. The Golden Rule was believed to be central to all of his teaching and should be practised 'all day and every day' (Armstrong, 2008).

The concept of compassion lies at the heart of most major religions, each of which have their own version of the Golden Rule requiring us to look into our hearts, identify what gives us pain and never inflict that pain on anyone else (Armstrong, 2008).

There has been some debate concerning the extent to which religion and/or spirituality drives compassion. A recent study identified that spirituality – beyond religiosity – may be uniquely associated with compassion and enhanced altruism (Saslow, et al., 2013) and it is argued that prosociality is driven to a greater extent by levels of compassion than religiosity (Saslow, et al., 2013). It is further suggested that although the relationship between religion and morality has long been debated, many scientific investigations have failed to decompose 'religion' and 'morality' into theoretically grounded elements and have neglected to consider the complex interplay between cognition and culture (McKay and Whitehouse, 2015). Religious and atheist individuals have diverging opinions regarding whether or not religion promotes altruism, and from a psychological perspective it would appear that there is a need to focus on people's specific emotions and behaviours in relation to altruism and the way in which these may influence or may be influenced by religion (Saroglou, 2013).

Compassion lies at the heart of most religious beliefs and practices, and since culture and religion impact on each other, it is important to understand these beliefs in the provision of culturally competent and compassionate healthcare. As such, the remainder of this chapter seeks to briefly look into the nature of compassion across five major religions.

Buddhism

Buddhism is largely based on the teachings of Gautama Buddha (c.563–c.483 BCE), known as 'the Buddha', and is a religion that encompasses a variety of traditions, beliefs and spiritual practices (Boardman, 2017).

Buddhist virtues and spiritual beliefs are closely linked to the concept of compassion and include qualities such as sharing and providing comfort, sympathy and concern. In addition, Buddhism realises that to feel for others, we need to feel for ourselves, and as such one's own spiritual development will develop naturally into concerns for others.

Indeed, this is demonstrated by the Buddha's own life, whereby after years of struggling for his own welfare, he was able to be of benefit to others (Dhammika, n.d.).

In the original Sanskrit Buddhist texts, the concept of compassion is described by the words *maitri* and *anukampa*. *Maitri* indicates a sense of fellowship with others, whilst *anukampa* represents a deep sense of empathy that arises during the encounter with suffering and leads to action (www.sgi.org/about-us/buddhist-concepts/compassion-solidarity-of-the-heart.html).

A key feature of the Buddhist spiritual life is that of 'enlightenment', the attainment of which represents the end of suffering. For enlightenment to be attained, Buddhist teachings state that a person is required to develop two qualities: wisdom and compassion (https://thebuddhistcentre.com/buddhism). Wisdom and compassion may be compared to two eyes that work together to see deeply, and these are the two key virtues of Buddhism (Mosig, 1989).

Shagdarsuren, Gerelmaa and Hamar (2016) suggest that Eastern medical ethics differ from Western medical ethics in so far as they consider the development of compassion to be a prerequisite to becoming a physician. In the traditional medicine of Tibet and Mongolia, a physician is viewed as an enlightened person who has been thoroughly trained in Buddhist philosophy. Thus, compassion is considered as a path to enlightenment and should be developed prior to entering the medical profession (Shagdarsuren, Gerelmaa and Hamar, 2016).

In traditions such as Buddhism, contemplation may often be used as a basis for the development of ethical consciousness (Mamgain, 2011). According to Mamgain (2011), the academic community should encourage this approach and assist students in the cultivation of a deep sense of ethical consciousness by using contemplative practices that lead to the development of heartfelt empathy and compassion.

In terms of healthcare, a critical review by Cheng and Tse (2015) has recently identified positive indicators in the use of Buddhist teachings in relation to mental health, including the four concepts of loving: kindness, compassion, empathetic joy and equanimity. Furthermore, Jormsri, et al. (2005) presented a model of moral competence in nursing utilising attributes founded on Thai culture. Moral competence was based on the Thai nursing value system and three dimensions were identified: moral perception, judgement and behaviour.

In 2016, Ahmadi, et al. (2016) conducted a study to explore the use of existential, spiritual and religious coping strategies among cancer patients in Korea. The study also aimed to investigate the impact of culture on patients' choice of coping methods. Four different coping strategies were identified: belief in the healing power of nature; the mind–body connection; relying on transcendent power; and finding oneself in relationships with others. These authors concluded by suggesting the importance of investigating cultural context when exploring the utilisation of meaning-making coping strategies in different countries.

Recently, the components of compassion have attracted interest from Western psychological science and research, and compassion is believed to represent a skill that one can train in. There is also increasing evidence that practising compassion can influence neurophysiological and immune systems (Gilbert, 2009). One focus of Buddhism that has become of particular interest to neuroscientists is that of the practice of meditation. Buddhist meditators report that the practice of calmly and mindfully observing the mental continuum results in a shift in the sense of self, and recently neuroscientists have conducted functional brain imaging studies focusing on contemplation (Kaszniak, 2010). Studies have demonstrated that expert Buddhist meditators have greater activation than meditation novices in empathy-related brain regions and that meditators who aim to benefit others rather than the self present with lower levels of depression, empathic distress and neuroticism (Kaszniak, 2010; O'Connor, et al., 2015).

Therapies deriving from Buddhist practices have become popular in modern-day psychotherapy. Closely related meditation practices include loving-kindness meditation (LKM) aimed at enhancing unconditional, positive emotional states of kindness and compassion (Hofmann, Grossman and Hinton, 2011). LKM represents a way of healing the troubled mind, thus freeing it from pain and confusion, and changing negative thoughts (Pannyavaro, n.d.). It is believed that LKM produces four qualities of love – friendliness, compassion, appreciative joy and equanimity – which naturally transforms into compassion as a result of an empathic response to other people (Pannyavaro, n.d.). Studies also support the positive effects of meditation and compassion interventions on a number of health outcomes, including healthcare provider burnout (Seppala, et al., 2014). Findings from a study by Seppala et al. (2014) suggest that LKM may represent a practical and time-effective solution for preventing burnout and promoting resilience in healthcare providers, thus improving quality of care in patients.

In addition, Hakan (2016) highlights a socio-existential dimension of mindfulness that may enhance social relationships and cultivate compassion among healthcare professionals, which may help them to improve their own health by overcoming the stress related to their work.

Shonin, Van Gordon and Griffiths (2014) report an increase in the scientific study of interventions that integrate Buddhist principles such as compassion and loving. These researchers sought to establish robust foundations for the clinical implementation of Buddhist principles by providing succinct and accurate interpretations of Buddhist terms and principles, an overview of current directions in the clinical operationalisation of Buddhist-derived interventions and an assessment of Buddhist-derived intervention clinical integration issues. The authors conclude that Buddhist-derived interventions may represent effective treatments for a variety of psychopathologies, but further research is needed.

SUMMARY

- Buddhist virtues and spiritual beliefs are closely linked to compassion.
- Buddhism realises that in order to feel for others, we need to feel for ourselves.
- According to Buddhist thought, one of the most powerful human desires is the desire for power over others, whereby the ego becomes most destructive.
- Buddhist teachings believe that a person should develop two qualities: wisdom and compassion.
- The ideal practice of Buddhism is to selflessly act to alleviate suffering.
- Of interest to neuroscientists is the Buddhist practice of meditation.
- It has been shown that expert Buddhist meditators have greater activation in empathy-related brain regions.
- Therapies emerging from Buddhist practices have become a popular subject.
- Meditation practice appears to encourage positive attitudes and emotional states of kindness and compassion.
- There is evidence that meditation can lead to greater compassion, in line with the beliefs of Buddhist theologians.

Islam

Islam is a religion founded by Muhammad, whose members worship the one God (Allah) of Jews and Christians and follow the teachings of the Koran (www.dictionary.com/browse/islam). Compassion is far more vital to Islamic teachings than anything else. In Islam, after the concepts of unity of God (*tawhid*) and *risalah* (the messengership of the Prophet Muhammad), compassion is believed to be as central to Islam as it is to Buddhism (Eusoff, 2010).

All except one of the 114 chapters of the Koran begin with the verse, "In the name of Allah the Compassionate, the Merciful." A good Muslim is to commence each day, each prayer and each significant action by invoking Allah the Merciful and Compassionate (www.newworldencyclopedia.org/entry/Virtue).

In relation to healthcare, Islamic bioethics is derived from a combination of principles, duties and rights. It emphasises prevention and teaches that the patient must be treated with respect and compassion. Also, the physical, mental and spiritual dimensions of the illness experience must all be taken into account (Daar and Al Khitamy, 2001). Halstead (2010) discusses the way in which most Muslims understand what is considered 'permitted' or 'forbidden' in terms of what God defines as right and good. Halstead suggests that moral education represents an inner change that is spiritual and comes about through the internalisation of universal Islamic values.

In terms of Islamic spiritual care, this involves a face-to-face individual interaction, representing a healing relationship between the patient and the spiritual caregiver. Islam regards both health and illness to emanate from God, closely linking the art of healing to worship (Fedorowicz and Walczyk, 2006). Marzband, Hosseini and Hamzehgardeshi (2016) suggest that the way in which spiritual care is defined may be influenced by the cultural and religious resources of the community. In their review of Islamic texts, the concept of spiritual care appeared to include a series of spiritual skills and competencies that help patients to achieve a good life.

Exploring nurse and patient experiences of spiritual care in Tabriz, Rassouli, et al. (2015) identified three categories: perceived barriers to providing spiritual care; communication; and religion-related spiritual experiences. It was reported that although nurses had few skills in responding to patients' spiritual needs, they remained a key source of energy, joy and hope for patients through their demonstration of empathy and compassion. Both patients and nurses utilised religious beliefs mentioned in Islam to strengthen patients' spiritual dimensions. These authors conclude that a framework should be provided to assist in the development of effective spiritual interventions that are sensitive to cultural differences (Rassouli, et al., 2015).

Furthermore, in a qualitative study by Atkinson (2015), the perceptions of the roles of Islamic values were explored among Muslim nurses in Kuwait. Nurses were interviewed and several key themes emerged. Among others, such themes included: altruistic relationships as a core value; all care as spiritual care; professional kinship that transcends culture, religion and nationality; and nursing ethics from divine ethics. The conclusions drawn indicate that the centrality of altruism in nursing care from the Islamic perspective and the integration of care of the spirit with care of the body are significant (Atkinson, 2015).

In developing codes of ethics for Iranian nurses, Shahriari, et al. (2015) extracted fifty-five ethical codes from twelve categories. The twelve categories were listed as: belief in human dignity; respect for patients' privacy; empathy for the patient; autonomy in decision-making; accurate and precise nursing care; being conscience; human relationships; professional commitment; promoting justice; preventing harm and/or injury; honesty and confidentiality; and maintaining and promoting professional values.

Recently, a further study was conducted by Zamanzadeh, et al. (2017) in an attempt to ascertain how compassionate care can be facilitated in daily practice from the perspective of Iranian nurses. A key theme emerged from this study, identified as 'deepening individual's capacity for compassionate care', and this consisted of three categories: personal system of values and beliefs; patient experience; and positive role models of compassion (Zamanzadeh, et al., (2017).

Babaei, Taleghani and Kayvanara (2016) stress the importance of understanding how compassion is demonstrated by nurses and how compassionate behaviour may differ across different cultures. Following a study with twenty nurses and twelve patients in six medical and four surgical wards in Iran, four cultural themes were elicited; love expression and compassion in the form of non-verbal emotional behaviours; empathy with others; emotional supports of patients at the bedside; and non-caring behaviours. These authors suggest that the results of this study could be of use to nurses, instructors and policy-makers. Furthermore, consideration of compassion in nursing and practical educational programmes and as an important component of patient-centred care is recommended (Babaei, Taleghani and Kayvanara, 2016).

SUMMARY

- Compassion is vital to Islamic teachings and represents the spirit of Islam.
- In the Muslim tradition, foremost among God's attributes are mercy and compassion.
- The Arabic word for compassion is 'rahmahm' and as a cultural influence its roots abound in the Koran.
- Islamic bioethics is derived from a combination of principles, duties and rights.
- Islamic bioethics teaches that the patient must be treated with respect and compassion.
- The physical, mental and spiritual dimensions of the illness experience must be taken into account.
- In terms of Islamic spiritual care, Muslim spiritual and religious caregivers are the main providers.
- The healing relationship of Muslim spiritual and religious caregivers with a client is an individual interaction based mainly on the therapeutic relationship.
- This represents a healing relationship between patients and the spiritual caregivers.

Hinduism

Hinduism is the world's third largest religion by population and is a religion or way of life found mainly in India and Nepal. With approximately one billion followers and with a 10,000-year history, Hinduism has been called the 'oldest religion' in the world. Scholars regard Hinduism as a fusion or synthesis of various Indian cultures and traditions, with diverse roots and no single founder (O'Doherty, 2017).

The virtue of showing compassion to all living beings is considered to be a central concept in Hindu philosophy (Kumar, 2014). Compassion as a virtue is governed and framed by the relational propriety dictated by *dharma*, the sacred order of the Hindu world. It is therefore difficult to differentiate compassion from service, charity, grace and social obligation, all of which may be expressions of compassion. There are three contexts for the Hindu notion of compassion, including yogic traditions of introspection, theistic traditions of devotion and the medieval compendia of *dharma* (http://what-when-how.com/love-in-world-religions/compassion-in-hinduism).

Detachment from the material world is thought to be achieved mainly through prayer and mantra meditation, although a number of other practices are included, such as congregational chanting and deity worship. It is believed that as one progresses, one starts to uncover the real nature of the soul together with qualities such as forgiveness, tolerance and kindness (Sachau, 1910).

The Hindu concepts of *karma* and *dharma* focus on unselfish action. The concept of *karma* is developed by caring for the poor and seeking good for others (Steffen and Masters, 2005). *Karma* refers to actions pertaining to the satisfaction of the body and mind, whereby every action is preceded by a stimulus and every action is followed by a reaction (Kang, 2010).

As reported by Jootun (2002), Hindu religious belief begins with the assumption that all living things have a soul that passes through cycles of birth and rebirth. Belief in *karma* is important to many Hindu patients, thus it is important for nurses to recognise the concepts of *karma* and rebirth.

Compassion has been considered as a virtue with many aspects, each explained by different terms. The most common terms include *daya*, *karuna* and *anukampa*. *Daya* is defined as the virtuous desire to mitigate the sorrow and difficulties of others by putting forth whatever effort necessary and as the value that treats all living beings as one's own self. Compassion to all living beings, including to those who are strangers and those who are foes, is seen as a noble virtue. *Karuna* refers to placing one's mind in another's position, thereby seeking to understand the other from their perspective. *Anukampa* refers to one's state after observing and understanding the pain and suffering in another (Balslev and Evers, 2009).

The ideals of Hinduism can be summarised into the word *ahimsa*, which represents the Hindu belief in love, care and compassion towards all living beings. *Ahimsa* extends beyond avoiding causing physical harm and also includes avoiding causing harm through speech and thought (Kemmerer and Nocella, 2011).

According to Hinduism, there are two forms of compassion: one for those who suffer even though they have done nothing wrong and one for those who suffer because they did something wrong. Absolute compassion applies to both, while relative compassion addresses the difference between the former and the latter. As claimed by Gandhi and others, the virtue of compassion to all living beings is a central concept in Hindu philosophy (https://en.wikipedia.org/wiki/Compassion#Hinduism).

Other words related to compassion in Hinduism include *karunya*, *ghrina*, *kripa* and *anukrosha*. Some of these words are used interchangeably among the schools of Hinduism to explain the concept of compassion, its sources, its consequences and its nature (Balslev and Evers, 2009).

There are many sources of Hindu thought that inspire men and women to live the ideals of compassion. The *rishis* who revealed the principles of *dharma* or divine law in Hindu scripture understood the potential for human suffering and how this could be avoided. To them, life was a coherent process leading all souls to enlightenment, and no violence could be carried to the higher reaches of that ascent (www.himalayanacademy.com/readlearn/basics/ahimsa-nonviolence).

In Hinduism, the person is viewed as a combination of mind, soul and body in the context of family, culture and environment, requiring a holistic approach to nursing interventions (Jootun, 2002). In matters of diagnosis and treatment, the senior elder and sometimes the extended family will often expect to be involved. Thus, it is vital for the nurse to involve the family while ensuring that the patient's wishes are respected (Jootun, 2002).

In 2007, Chattopadhyay reported on the surge of interest in understanding the interaction of religion, spirituality, health and medicine and the fact that many studies suggest that religious practice is associated with better physical and mental health outcomes. Chattopadhyay (2007) suggests that this interest in the interaction of religion and spirituality with health and medicine has significant implications within an Indian context. Understanding and acknowledging the spiritual needs of patients may help in the development of ensuring that care is holistic, ethical and compassionate (Chattopadhyay, 2007).

Belief in *karma* and reincarnation feature strongly in Hinduism, and it is believed that any thought, feeling or action portrayed from one to another will return to the originator. There is a belief that what we do to others will be done to us, if not in this life then in another. Almost all Hindus are influenced by the concept of *karma*, which can assist the individual in coming to terms with life events and help them to move forward. Every form of illness, whether physical or mental, is understood to have a biological, psychological and spiritual component. As such, treatment that includes all three areas is considered to be the most effective (Kang, 2010).

SUMMARY

- Hinduism has been referred to as the 'oldest religion' in the world.
- The virtue of compassion is considered to be a central concept in Hinduism.
- Compassion to all living beings, including strangers, is seen as a noble virtue.
- Compassion as a virtue is governed and framed by the relational propriety dictated by *dharma* – the sacred order of the Hindu world.
- Compassion is considered to be a virtue with many strands, each explained by different terms.
- The most common terms include *daya*, *karuna* and *anukampa*.
- Compassion is feeling at one with the sufferer and is the basis for *ahimsa*, a core virtue in Hinduism.
- In Hinduism, there are two forms of compassion: one for those who suffer even though they have done nothing wrong and one for those who suffer because they did something wrong.
- Absolute compassion applies to both of the above, while relative compassion addresses the difference between the former and the latter.

Judaism

Judaism was founded over 3500 years ago in the Middle East and is one of the oldest mono-theistic religions. Jewish people believe that God appointed them to be his chosen people in order to set an example of holiness and ethical behaviour to the world (www.bbc.co.uk/religion/religions/judaism/).

Compassion in Judaism is one of the central attributes of the divine and one of the core obligations of humanity. The Hebrew Bible describes God as both compassionate and merciful (http://what-when-how.com/love-in-world-religions/compassion-in-judaism/). Judaism teaches involvement and concern with the plight of fellow human beings. Every life is sacred, and there is an obligation to do whatever can be done to help others (Schwartz, n.d.).

In the Jewish tradition, God is invoked as the Father of Compassion. Sorrow and pity for one in distress, creating a desire to relieve it in view of the sufferer's helplessness, is essential to Judaism. The Biblical conception of compassion is the feeling of the parent for the child.

A classic articulation of the Golden Rule came from the first century Rabbi Hillel the Elder, renowned as one of the most important figures in Jewish history. Asked for a summary of the Jewish religion in the most concise terms, Hillel stated: "That which is hateful to you, do not do to your fellow. That is the whole Torah. The rest is the explanation; go and learn" (www.all-creatures.org/cap/comp-judaism.shtml). The Jewish people have a highly moral lifestyle and regard the Jewish Bible (the Torah) and its commandments and teachings as a way of life rather than a religion (Collins, 2002).

As reported by Prince (2009), implicit within Judaism is a vision of human well-being that is grounded in a fierce engagement with life, the importance of community and a belief that sacred texts and rituals can be relevant to modern dilemmas. It is both an intensely private experience and inextricably bound to the fate of the collective. The field of Judaism, health, and healing draws on a deeply rooted wisdom with regard to the effects of stress, isolation, loss, hard times and celebration on the body, mind and spirit (Prince, 2009).

Rosner (2004) reported that the Jewish people generally have a negative view towards full disclosure of a fatal illness to a patient. This is because of the fear that the patient may give up hope, suffer severe mental anguish, become despondent and die sooner than otherwise. Shortening a patient's life is strictly forbidden because Judaism espouses the concept that God-given life is sacred. Disclosure should therefore be made within the context of optimism. The most positive outlook should be imparted to the patient, and this should be performed with compassion and hope (Rosner, 2004). Likewise, as reported by Baider (2012), families may be reluctant to disclose the diagnosis of a terminal illness because of the belief that this may lead to emotional trauma for the patient or premature death.

As reported by Goldsand, Rosenberg and Gordon (2001), Jewish bioethics emerged from the practice of applying principles of Jewish law to ethical dilemmas. Interpretation of foundational texts such as the Bible and the Talmud may help to clarify the duties of physicians and patients when difficult healthcare decisions arise. These authors put forward the view that although Jewish law is an integral consideration of religiously observant Jews, secularised Jewish patients often welcome the wisdom of their tradition when considering treatment options (Goldsand, Rosenberg and Gordon, 2001).

In a study to examine perceptions of cancer and cancer screening and to identify ways to promote screening among ultra-orthodox women (Freund, Cohen and Azaiza, 2014), three main themes emerged: faith in God; the Rabbi as a guide; and one's relationship with the community. These researchers suggest that the findings from this study highlight the importance of studying the specific needs of members of certain religious groups, as the knowledge gained may guide them to provide the most appropriate compassionate care.

Shabtai, Pirutinsky and Rosmarin (2015) propose the integration of Jewish spiritual beliefs into the use of standard cognitive behavioural therapy for various mental health disorders. It is reported that such integration may provide an effective (and compassionate) path towards cognitive and behavioural change and that drawing upon psychological insights within the Jewish tradition may be effective for individuals from other faiths, in addition to those from the Jewish faith (Shabtai, Pirutinsky and Rosmarin, 2015).

Judaism provides a vision for compassionate care throughout the continuum of illness – from sickness and death to grieving and mourning. The traditions span centuries and the rituals remain relevant in contemporary society. These practices have meaning for those immersed in Jewish faith and culture and provide lessons for others (https://divinity.duke.edu/sites/divinity.duke.edu/files/documents/tmc/Jewish-Ritual.pdf).

SUMMARY

- Jewish people believe that God appointed them to be his chosen people in order to set an example of holiness and ethical behaviour to the world.
- Compassion in Judaism is one of the core obligations of humanity.
- Judaism teaches involvement and concern with the plight of fellow human beings.
- Every life is sacred, and there is an obligation to do whatever can be done to help others.

- Jewish people have a highly moral lifestyle and regard the Jewish Bible (the Torah) and its teachings as a way of life rather than a religion.
- The field of Judaism, health and healing draws on a deeply rooted wisdom.
- Judaism has much to say about the effects of stress, isolation, loss, hard times and celebration on the body, mind and spirit.
- The Jewish people generally have a negative view towards full disclosure of a fatal illness to a patient because of the fear that the patient may give up hope.
- Judaism provides a vision for compassionate care throughout the continuum of illness – from sickness and death to grieving and mourning.

Christianity

For Christians, the life of Jesus embodies the very essence of compassion and relational care, and his example challenges Christians to forsake their own desires and to act compassionately towards others, particularly those in need or distress (www.la.utexas.edu/users/bump/Compassion/Compassion%20overview.htm).

The term 'Christian values' historically refers to the values derived from the teachings of Jesus and taught by Christians throughout the history of the religion (Kurian and Lamport, 2015).

Christian values are based on God and the teachings of Jesus Christ, with the most important value being to value God more than anything, anybody or any idea. Christian values are spiritual in nature, but the values are evidenced through deeds and actions. Core Christian values include hope, righteousness, love and putting God first (http://access-jesus.com/christian-values-html/).

In the Sermon on the Mount, Jesus assures his listeners that "Blessed are the merciful, for they shall obtain mercy." In the Parable of the Good Samaritan, he holds up to his followers the ideal of compassionate conduct. True Christian compassion, say the Gospels, should extend to all, even to the extent of loving one's enemies (www.all-creatures.org/cap/comp-christianity.shtml).

Within the Christian Bible's Second Epistle to the Corinthians, God is spoken of as the "Father of compassion" and the "God of all comfort." It reads:

> Praise be to the God and Father of our Lord Jesus Christ, the Father of compassion and the God of all comfort, who comforts us in all our troubles, so that we can comfort those in any trouble with the comfort we ourselves received from God. For just as the sufferings of Christ flow over into our lives, so also through Christ our comfort overflows. If we are distressed, it is for your comfort and salvation; if we are comforted, it is for your comfort, which produces in you patient endurance of the same sufferings we suffer. And our hope for you is firm, because we know that just as you share in our sufferings, so also you share in our comfort.
>
> *(www.all-creatures.org/cap/comp-christianity.shtml)*

For the Christian, suffering is not necessarily meaningless, and it can be seen as redemptive. For a Christian to share the suffering of another means that he/she may bring light into that person's life (Demarco, n.d.).

Within Christianity, hospitality is the imperative of welcoming the stranger to our table (Arrington, 2017). As such, Arrington (2017) suggests that a hospitality framework may be helpful for the development of world Christians. It is suggested that hospitality as a framework can help to cultivate empathy through listening and learning and engender transformation because it forces us to leave familiar structures and view life through the eyes of the other (Arrington, 2017).

In Christianity, Jesus is believed to have exemplified all of the Father's attributes, including compassion. Moved with compassion for the suffering of others, Jesus healed the large crowds who came to him (Matthew 14:14), and when asked what was the greatest commandment, Jesus responded that it is to love God with all our heart, mind and strength. But he added that the second commandment is 'Love your neighbour as yourself'. The Bible is clear that compassion is an attribute of God and of God's people as well (www.gotquestions.org/Bible-compassion.html).

In Greek Orthodoxy, it has been said that:

> The word of God tells us that our role in terms of us and others is one, to love and have compassion: Owe no one anything except to love one another, for he who loves another has fulfilled the law.

And that:

> Those that love and have compassion do not miss out, they get back a lot more than what they give.
>
> *(www.greekorthodox.org.au)*

Throughout both the Old and New Testaments, Christians are commanded to imitate God's compassion for others. The call in the Bible to embody the compassion of God is so strong that it is equated with knowing God. Many Christians speak of a personal relationship with God that provides meaning, purpose and joy to those who enter into it. According to the Bible, to know God is to defend the cause of the poor and needy and to live out the life of Jesus Christ, in whom the fullness of God was pleased to dwell (www.worldvision.com.au/docs/default-source/our-christian-identity/wva_oci_compassion_of_christ.pdf?sfvrsn=2).

Sulmasy (2016) suggests that with a growth in the interests in medicine and religion, a more explicit 'witnessing' by Christian physicians may be required. This author puts forward suggestions based on linguistic, scriptural and theological reflection with regard to the way in which physicians and the Church may both witness Christ and give witness to Christ in the care of the sick, offering a new insight into what it means to witness and to heal as Christian.

Within Christianity, medical compassion has been defined as a physician's deliberate act or habit of explicitly observing a suffering person and relating to that patient with '*agape*', the term Christians used to describe love and compassion (Guinan, 2014).

Christ challenges Christians to forsake their own desires and to act compassionately towards others, particularly those in need or distress. According to the Gospels, true Christian compassion should extend to all, including loving one's enemies (http://habiartfoundation.org/global-compassion.aspx).

The Christian morality associated with the early days of nursing relates to the character training of nurses advocated by Florence Nightingale. She was in no doubt that nurses needed to bring science, technical knowledge, skills and evidence to the task of caring for patients, together with empathy and compassion (Maben, Cornwell and Sweeny, 2009)

In nineteenth-century Great Britain, Christianity was the prominent religion, advocating that followers should always be compassionate in their deeds and actions (Straughair, 2012). Florence Nightingale was a Christian who translated her ideals into the characterisation of the professional nurse, famously portraying the image of the ministering angel performing the work of God (Straughair, 2012).

SUMMARY

- For Christians, the life of Jesus embodies the very essence of compassion.
- In the Parable of the Good Samaritan, Jesus holds up to his followers the ideal of compassionate conduct.
- According to the Gospels, true Christian compassion should extend to all, even to the extent of loving one's enemies.
- In Christianity, Jesus is believed to have exemplified all of the Father's attributes, including compassion.
- The Bible is clear that compassion is an attribute of God and of God's people as well.
- Throughout both the Old and New Testaments, Christians are commanded to imitate God's compassion for others.
- According to the Bible, to know God is to defend the cause of the poor and needy and to live out the life of Jesus Christ.
- In nineteenth-century Great Britain, Christianity was the prominent religion, advocating that followers should always be compassionate in their deeds and actions.
- Florence Nightingale was a Christian who translated her ideals into the characterisation of the professional nurse, famously portraying the image of the ministering angel performing the work of God.

Concluding remarks

As outlined above, compassion clearly features highly in all major religions, being at the core of most faiths and a concept upon which many religious doctrines seem to be based.

However, whilst the concept of compassion is historically and traditionally embedded into all major religions, there remains some debate as to how this translates into behaviour. We can observe certain measurable effects of Buddhist meditation practice on compassionate behaviour via neuroscience, but some studies question the extent to which compassionate care may be influenced by religion/spirituality or may influence religion/spirituality (Saslow, et al., 2013). Within this light, it has been suggested that altruism is an important, but not unique, psychological dimension of religion. Well-being, moral integrity and social cohesion and individuation are also important dimensions of religion. Understanding how these dimensions are affected by or shape religious prosociality remains an issue to be fully investigated (Saroglou, 2013).

The study of different religions can assist in the attainment of a more accurate knowledge of patients' religious beliefs and practices, providing an opportunity for healthcare providers to more adequately meet the needs of their patients (Bursey, 2010).

Understanding the link between compassion and religion and how this is integrated into different religious/cultural groups can be important in facilitating culturally competent and compassionate healthcare.

LEARNING ACTIVITIES

- Write a few notes to compare and contrast the compassion principles of two of the major religions discussed within this chapter.
- Write some notes on how you think an understanding of different religions, beliefs and practices can enhance your efforts to provide culturally competent and compassionate healthcare.
- Write a couple of sentences on your own beliefs and personal values that might help you cope with any problems you may face in life by practicing self-compassion.
- Explain the extent to which you feel your own personal beliefs influence your beliefs about compassionate healthcare.
- Write a very brief story or poem reflecting your own or another person's experience whereby religious, spiritual and/or personal beliefs have influenced you either as a care-receiver or a caregiver.

References

Access-Jesus (n.d.). What are Christian Values? Retrieved from: http://access-jesus.com/christian-values–html.

Ahmadi, F., Park, J., Kim, K.M. and Ahmadi, N. (2016). Exploring existential coping resources: The perspective of Koreans with cancer. *Journal of Religion and Health*, 55(6), pp. 2053–2068.

All-Creatures (n.d.). Compassion Actions Project – Judaism. Retrieved from: www.all-creatures.org/cap/comp-judaism.shtml.

All-Creatures (n.d.). Views on compassion – christianity. Retrieved April 2016 from: www.all-creatures.org/cap/comp-christianity.shtml.

Armstrong, K. (2008). Do unto others. *The Guardian*. Retrieved from: www.theguardian.com/commentisfree/2008/nov/14/religion.

Arrington, A. (2017). Becoming a world Christian: Hospitality as a framework for engaging Otherness. *International Journal of Christianity and Education*, 21(1), pp. 26–38.

Atkinson, C. (2015). Islamic values and nursing practice in Kuwait. *Journal of Holistic Nursing*, 33(3), pp. 195–204.

Babaei, S., Taleghani, F. and Kayvanara, M. (2016). Compassionate behaviours of clinical nurses in Iran: An ethnographic study. *International Nursing Review*. Retrieved from http://onlinelibrary.wiley.com/doi/10.1111/inr.12296/full.

Baider, L. (2012). Cultural diversity: Family path through terminal illness. *Annals of Oncology*, 23(3), pp. 62–65.

Balslev, A. and Evers, D., eds (2009). *Compassion in the world's religions: Envisioning human solidarity*. Munster, Germany, LIT Verlag.

BAPS (n.d.). Spiritual Living. Retrieved June 2016 from: www.baps.org/Spiritual-Living/Hindu-Beliefs/Compassion-and-Nonviolence-Ahimsa.aspx.

BBC (n.d.). Hinduism. Retrieved from: www.bbc.co.uk/religion/religions/hinduism.

BBC (n.d.). Judaism. Retrieved from: www.bbc.co.uk/religion/religions/judaism.

Boardman, J.E. (2017). *Ordained before the world: A Catholic apologetic.* Raleigh, NC: The Goldhead Group.

The Buddhist Centre (n.d.). Buddhism for today. Retrieved April 2016 from: https://thebuddhistcentre.com/buddhism.

Bursey, E. (2010). Introduction. In: S. Sorajjakool, M.F. Carr and J.J. Nam, eds. *World religions for healthcare professionals.* New York, Oxon: Routledge, pp. 1–14.

Chattopadhyay, S. (2007). Religion, spirituality, health and medicine: Why should Indian physicians care? *Journal of Postgraduate Medicine,* 53(4), pp. 262–266.

Cheng, F.K. and Tse, S. (2015). Applying the Buddhist four immeasurables to mental health care: A critical review. *Journal of Religion and Spirituality in Social Work: Social Thought,* 34(1), pp. 24–50.

Collins, A. (2002). Nursing with dignity part 1: Judaism. *Nursing Times.* Retrieved from: www.nursingtimes.net/roles/nurse-managers/nursing-with-dignity-part-1-judaism/205662.fullarticle.

Daar, A.S. and Al Khitamy, A.B. (2001). Bioethics for clinicians: 21. Islamic bioethics. *CMAJ,* 164(1), pp. 60–63.

Demarco, D. (n.d.). The virtue of compassion. Retrieved February 2017 from: www.catholiceducation.org/en/culture/catholic-contributions/the-virtue-of-compassion.html.

Dhammika, V.S. (n.d.). Wisdom and compassion. Retrieved April 2016 from: www.buddhanet.net/e-learning/qanda07.htm.

Dictionary.com (n.d.). Islam. Retrieved from: www.dictionary.com/browse/islam.

Eusoff, S. (2010). The centrality of compassion In Islam. Speech given at The Sea Of Faith Conference, Wellington, New Zealand. Retrieved June 2016 from: www.iman.co.nz/sultan_compassion_speech.php.

Fedorowicz, S. and Walczyk T.C. (2006). A trisomial concept of sociocultural and religious factors in healthcare decision-making and service provision in the Muslim Arab world. In: I. Papadopoulos, ed. *Transcultural health and social care: Development of culturally competent practitioners.* Edinburgh, UK: Churchill Livingstone Elsevier, pp. 265–283.

Freund, A., Cohen, M. and Azaiza, F. (2014). The doctor is just a messenger: Beliefs of ultraorthodox Jewish women in regard to breast cancer and screening. *Journal of Religion and Health,* 53(4), pp. 1075–1090.

Gilbert, P. (2009). Introducing compassion-focused therapy. *Advances in Psychiatric Treatment,* 15(3), pp. 199–208.

Goldsand, G., Rosenberg, Z.R.S. and Gordon, M. (2001). Bioethics for clinicians: 22 Jewish bioethics. *CMAJ,* 164(2), pp. 219–222.

Gotquestions.org (n.d.). What does the Bible say about compassion? Retrieved April 2016 from: www.gotquestions.org/Bible-compassion.html.

Guinan, P. (2014). Faith in medicine. Compassion in medicine. *Catholic Medical Quarterly,* 64(1). Retrieved from: www.cmq.org.uk/CMQ/2014/Feb/compassion_in_medicine.html.

Hakan, N. (2016). Socioexistential mindfulness: Bringing empathy and compassion into health care practice. *Spirituality in Clinical Practice,* 3(1), pp. 22–31.

Halstead, J.M. (2010). Islamic values: A distinctive framework for moral education? *Journal of Moral Education,* 36(3), pp. 283–296.

Hofmann, S.G., Grossman, P. and Hinton, D.E. (2011). Loving-kindness and compassion meditation: Potential for psychological interventions. *Clinical Psychology Review,* 31(7), pp. 1126–1132.

Duke Divinity School (2007). Jewish Ritual, Reality and Response at the end of Life. Retrieved May 2016 from: https://divinity.duke.edu/sites/divinity.duke.edu/files/documents/tmc/Jewish-Ritual.pdf.

Jootun, D. (2002). Nursing with dignity. *Nursing Times,* 98(15), p.38.

Jormsri, P., Kunaviktikul, W., Ketefian, S. and Chaowalit, A. (2005). Moral competence in nursing practice. *Nursing Ethics,* 12(6), pp. 582–594.

Kang, C. (2010). Hinduism and mental health: Engaging British Hindus. *Mental Health, Religion & Culture*, 13(6), pp. 587–593.

Kaszniak, A.W. (2010). Empathy and compassion in Buddhism and neuroscience. Retrieved June 2016 from: www.pbs.org/thebuddha/blog/2010/Mar/17/empathy-and-compassion-buddhism-and-neuroscience-a.

Kauai's Hindu Monastery (n.d.). Basics of Hinduism – The Hindu ethic of non-violence. Retrieved May 2016 from: www.himalayanacademy.com/readlearn/basics/ahimsa-nonviolence.

Kemmerer, L. and Nocella, A. (2011). *Call to compassion*. New York, NY: Lantern Books.

Kumar, S. (2014). Compassion: Elixir of life. Retrieved June 2017 from: www.speakingtree.in/blog/compassion-elixir-of-life.

Kurian, G.T. and Lamport, M.A. (2015). *Encyclopedia of Christian education*, Vol.3, p.1337. Lanham, MD: Rowman & Littlefield.

Maben J., Cornwell J. and Sweeney K. (2009). In praise of compassion. *Journal of Research in Nursing*, 15(1), pp. 9–13.

Mamgain, V. (2011). Ethical consciousness in the classroom: How Buddhist practices can help develop empathy and compassion. *Journal of Transformative Education*, 8(1), pp. 22–41.

Marzband, R., Hosseini, S.H. and Hamzehgardeshi, Z. (2016). A concept analysis of spiritual care based on Islamic sources. *Religions*, 7(6), p.61.

McKay, R. and Whitehouse, H. (2015). Religion and morality. *Psychological Bulletin*, 141(2), pp. 447–473.

Mosig, Y.D. (1989). Wisdom and compassion: What the Buddha taught a psycho-poetical analysis. *Theoretical & Philosophical Psychology*, 9(2), pp. 27–36.

New World Encyclopedia (n.d.). Virtue. Retrieved from: www.newworldencyclopedia.org/entry/Virtue.

O'Connor, L.E., Rangan, R.K., Berry, J.W., Stiver, D.J., Hanson, R., Ark, A. and Li, T. (2015). Empathy, compassionate altruism and psychological well-being in contemplative practitioners across five traditions. *Psychology*, 6(8), pp. 989–1000.

O'Doherty, M. (2017). *Reconciling religion and human rights in the information age*. Crystal Grove Books.

Pannyavaro, V. (n.d.). Loving kindness meditation. Retrieved May 2016 from: www.buddhanet.net/e-learning/loving-kindness.htm.

Prince, M.F. (2009). Judaism, health, and healing: How a new Jewish communal field took root and where it might grow. *Journal of Jewish Communal Service*, 84(3/4), pp. 280–291.

Rassouli, M., Zamanzahdeh, V., Ghahramanian, A., Abbazadeh, A., Alavi-Majd, H. and Nikanfar, A. (2015). Experiences of patients with cancer and their nurses on the conditions of spiritual care and spiritual interventions in oncology units. *Iranian Journal of Nursing and Midwidery Research*, 20(1), pp. 25–33.

Rosner, F. (2004). Informing the patient about a fatal disease: From paternalism to autonomy – The Jewish view. *Cancer Investigation*, 22(6), pp. 949–953.

Sachau, E.C. (1910). *Alberuni's India. An account of the religion, philosophy, literature, geography, chronology, astronomy, customs, laws and astrology of India*. Vol.1. London, UK: Kegan Paul, Trench, Trubner and Co. Ltd.

Saroglou, V. (2013). Religion, spirituality, and altruism. In: *APA handbook of psychology, religion, and spirituality: Vol. 1. Context, theory, and research*, Washington, DC: APA, Ch.24, pp. 1–20.

Saslow, L.R., John, O.P., Piff, P.K., Willer, R. Wong, E., Impett, E.A., Kogan, A., Antonenko, O., Clark, K., Feinberg, M., Keltner, D. and Saturn, S.R. (2013). The social significance of spirituality: New perspectives on the compassion–altruism relationship. *Psychology of Religion and Spirituality*, 5(3), pp. 201–218.

Saslow, L.R., Willer, R., Feinber, M., Piff, P.K., Clark, K., Keltner, D. and Saturn, S.R. (2013). My brother's keeper? Compassion predicts generosity more among less religious individuals. *Social Psychological and Personality Science*, 4(1), pp. 31–38.

Schwartz, R. (n.d.). Issues in Jewish ethics: The Jewish response to hunger. Retrieved May 2016 from: www.jewishvirtuallibrary.org/jsource/Judaism/hunger.html.

Seppala, E.M., Hutcherson, C.A., Nguyen, D.T.H., Doty, J.R. and Gross, J.J. (2014). Loving-kindness meditation: A tool to improve healthcare provider compassion, resilience, and patient care. *Journal of Compassionate Health Care (Open Access)*. Retrieved from: http://jcompassionatehc.biomedcentral. com/articles/10.1186/s40639-014-0005-9.

SGI (2010). Compassion: Solidarity of the Heart SGI quarterly. Retrieved May 2016 from: www.sgi. org/about-us/buddhism-in-daily-life/compassion-solidarity-of-the-heart.html.

Shabtai, D.G., Pirutinsky, S. and Rosmarin, D.H. (2015). Integrating Judaism into cognitive behavioral therapy. In: M. Ben-Avie, Y. Ives and K. Loewenthal, eds. *Applied Jewish values in social sciences and psychology*. Cham, Switzerland: Springer, pp. 133–151.

Shagdarsuren, D., Gerelmaa, B. and Hamar, D. (2016). Compassion in medical ethics of traditional Mongolian medicine. *Asian Bioethics Review*, 8(4), pp. 302–306.

Shahriari, M., Mohammadi, E., Fooladi, M.M., Abbaszadeh, A. and Bahrami, M. (2015). Proposing codes of ethics for Iranian nurses. *Journal of Mixed Methods Research*, 10(4), pp. 352–366.

Shonin, E., Van Gordon, W. and Griffiths, M.D. (2014). The emerging role of Buddhism in clinical psychology: Toward effective integration. *Psychology of Religion and Spirituality*, 6(2), pp. 123–137.

Steffen, P.R. and Masters, K.S. (2005). Does compassion mediate the intrinsic religion–health relationship? *Annals of Behavioral Medicine*, 30(3), pp. 217–224.

Straughair, C. (2012). Exploring compassion: Implications for contemporary nursing. Part 1. *British Journal of Nursing*, 21(3), pp. 160–164.

Sulmasy, D.P. (2016). Christian witness in health care. *Christian Bioethics*, 22(1), pp. 45–61.

What-When-How (n.d.). Compassion in Hinduism. Retrieved May 2016 from: http://what-when-how.com/love-in-world-religions/compassion-in-hinduism.

What-When-How (n.d.). Compassion in Judaism. Retrieved July 2016 from: http://what-when-how. com/love-in-world-religions/compassion-in-judaism.

Wikipedia (n.d.). Compassion and Hinduism. Retrieved from: https://en.wikipedia.org/wiki/ Compassion#Hinduism.

Wikipedia (n.d.). Compassion. Retrieved from: www.la.utexas.edu/users/bump/Compassion/ Compassion%20overview.htm.

Wikipedia (n.d.). Hindu Ethics. Retrieved from: https://en.wikipedia.org/wiki/Ethics_in_ religion#Hindu_ethics.

World Vision Australia (n.d.). Our Christian identity. Retrieved June 2016 from: www.worldvision.com. au/docs/default-source/our-christian-identity/wva_oci_compassion_of_christ.pdf?sfvrsn=2.

Zamanzadeh, V., Valizadeh, L., Rahmani, A., van der Cingel, M. and Ghafourifard, M. (2017). Factors facilitating nurses to deliver compassionate care: A qualitative study. *Scandinavian Journal of Caring Sciences*. Retrieved from: http://onlinelibrary.wiley.com/doi/10.1111/scs.12434/full.

4

HEALTH AND ILLNESS IN MULTICULTURAL SOCIETIES[1]

Introduction

All human beings are cultural beings. Culture is the shared way of life of a group of people that includes beliefs, values, ideas, language, communication, norms and visibly expressed forms such as customs, art, music, clothing and etiquette. Culture influences individuals' lifestyles, personal identities and their relationships with others both within and outside their culture. Cultures are dynamic and ever changing as individuals are influenced by and influence their culture by different degrees (Papadopoulos, 2006).

Fundamental to an understanding of health and illness in multicultural societies is the realisation that different cultural and ethnic groups may differ in their healthcare values, beliefs and behaviours. For care to be culturally competent, a number of factors need to be taken into consideration, including self-awareness, similarities and differences, cultural identity, trust, respect and health inequalities. This chapter aims to briefly explore factors relating to personal values, cultural identity, 'otherness' and socio-cultural determinants of health before introducing the Papadopoulos, Tilki and Taylor (PTT) model of cultural competence (Papadopoulos, 2006), the values and principles of which are derived from the body of knowledge around human rights, transcultural ethics, health inequalities, migration, intercultural relations and communication, socio-political systems, human caring and compassion.

Personal values

Unique to being human is the fact that as individuals we all hold our own personal beliefs, values and attitudes, which develop throughout the course of our lives and may be influenced by a number of factors including family, friends, community, life experience and religion. If we compare what we value with a friend or fellow student who comes from a different cultural background to ours, we will soon discover that we have much in common. For example, we may discover that we both value love, life, justice, family life, health and so on. We will, however, discover that our interpretations and expressions of love, life, justice, family life and health differ to some degree (Papadopoulos, 2006).

Within the healthcare setting, we may interact with many individuals from different cultural or religious backgrounds. As such, we need to be aware of our own personal beliefs and values and the impact they may have on our relationships with those we care for and their families.

It is important to always consider the personal beliefs of patients, even though according to the General Medical Council (GMC) some beliefs of patients may lead them to ask for a procedure for religious, cultural or social reasons or refuse treatment that healthcare professionals consider to be of overall benefit to them (www.gmc-uk.org/guidance/ethical_guidance/21179.asp). The standard 'Treat people as individuals' within the Nursing and Midwifery Council (NMC) Code states that we must not discriminate in any way against those in our care. Nurses practise in diverse cultural environments and should always take care not to offend patients' values and beliefs (Orford, 2012). However, we may from time to time have to challenge such beliefs. One example is the belief by members of some cultural groups that young girls should be circumcised (i.e. female genital mutilation).

Personal beliefs and values may be seen as the starting points for morality and ethics, which are acquired over time from a variety of sources. Values may represent the beliefs, qualities and principles held in high regard by both individuals and groups. Values help to guide our lives on a personal and professional level and can also be instrumental in decision-making.

In a study designed to measure professional and personal values among nurses and to identify the factors affecting these values, 323 Israeli nurses were asked to rate thirty-six personal values and twenty professional values. The top ten rated values were predominantly concerned with nurses' responsibilities towards patients. The values of human dignity, equality among patients and prevention of suffering were rated as most important. For personal values, honesty and responsibility were rated first. As reported by these researchers, such findings may assist us in understanding the motives of nurses with different characteristics and help to promote their work according to professional ethical values (Rassin, 2008).

Health and illness

Health refers to a state of well-being that is culturally defined, valued and practised and that reflects the ability of individuals (or groups) to perform their daily activities in culturally expressed, beneficial and patterned lifeways (Leininger, 1991). Illness refers to an unwanted condition that is culturally defined and culturally responded to (Papadopoulos, 2006).

Western societies may view disease as a result of natural 'scientific' phenomena and encourage the use of technology to diagnose and treat disease. Other societies, including indigenous groups, may believe that illness is the result of supernatural phenomena and may promote a range of cultural practices, as well as prayer or other spiritual interventions (McLaughlin and Braun, 1998). Thus, culturally shaped notions of health and illness may have a strong impact on how individuals engage in help-seeking and how they view service use (Campbell and Long, 2014).

An immensely necessary component in the formation of the nurse–patient relationship is that of communication. To achieve effective therapeutic communication is challenging, but this can be aided if nurses and other healthcare providers understand the impact that culture has on their patients' values, beliefs and practices. In doing so, healthcare professionals will conclude that patient engagement enables them to compare their own health and illness beliefs and values with those of their patients and/or their families, to consider the similarities and differences and to reach a culturally acceptable and beneficial compromise. This is a most important step towards providing culturally competent and compassionate care that promotes health and alleviates illness.

SUMMARY

- Culture is the shared way of life of a group of people that includes beliefs, values and ideas.
- As individuals, we all hold our own personal beliefs, values and attitudes that develop throughout the course of our lives.
- Values may be referred to as the beliefs, qualities or principles that an individual or group of people hold in high regard.
- Within the healthcare setting, we may interact with many individuals from different cultural or religious backgrounds.
- It is important to realise that different cultural and ethnic groups may differ in their healthcare values, beliefs and behaviours.
- Culturally shaped notions of health and illness may have a strong impact on how individuals engage in help-seeking and how they view service use.
- Nurses should understand their own worldviews, beliefs and value systems in order to be able to better understand and respect those of their clients.
- Therapeutic communication is challenging, but this can be aided if nurses understand the impact that culture has on their patients' values, beliefs and practices.

Cultural identity

Even though all human beings have much in common, our small or subtle differences are important, as they are the ones that define our uniqueness and our individuality (Papadopoulos, 2006). Our individuality is closely linked to the notion of personal identity, which is also influenced by many factors. For example, important components of my identity are my gender (a woman), my marital status (a wife), my family status (a mother, a grandmother), my politics (for democracy, equality and human rights), my ethnicity (a first-generation migrant Greek Cypriot), my religion (Christianity) and my job status (an academic).

Understanding the significance of cultural identity is essential for developing cultural competence. Cultural identity refers to the feeling of belonging to a group and is part of a person's self-conception relating to factors such as nationality, ethnicity, religion and social class.

According to Adler (2002), the concept of cultural identity can be used in two different ways. First, it can be employed as a reference to the collective self-awareness that a given group embodies and reflects, together with their shared values, beliefs and cultural behaviours. A second use of the concept concerns the identity of the individual in relation to his or her culture. The concept of cultural identity is considered to be a fundamental symbol of a person's existence and sense of self that is dependent on stability of values and a sense of wholeness and integration.

Kung, et al. (2016) report that cultural differences in beliefs about the fixedness of the world promote different intuitions about identity continuity. These authors suggest that people from a society with rigid social systems should perceive more identity discontinuity when a person's social relationships change, whereas those from a society with more flexible social systems should perceive the reverse. In testing this hypothesis by comparing fixed-world beliefs and perceptions of identity discontinuity in India and the USA, the authors identified that Indians perceive more identity discontinuity than Americans when relationships change, which may be explained by Indians' stronger fixed-world beliefs.

Furthermore, understanding cultural identity may have implications for mental healthcare. It is reported that the governing bodies for psychiatry, psychology and social work all support culturally competent mental healthcare and have called for increased awareness of the importance of racial, ethnic and cultural identity in mental health treatment and outcomes (Hack, et al., 2014). In addition, research with asylum seekers and refugees in mental healthcare suggests utilising the importance of cultural identity as a way to explore the meanings of illness and the interrelationship between the patient and healthcare provider (Groen, 2009). Groen states that it is essential to gain the trust of and 'recognise' the patient, and that this could possibly be achieved via a cultural interview in which cultural references of the healthcare provider and the patient are exchanged (Groen, 2009).

Differences in patient–provider perceptions in terms of ill health and treatment options have been associated with poor patient outcomes. In a study by Garroutte, et al. (2006), the extent to which healthcare providers and American–Indian patients disagreed on patient health status ratings and how such differences related to patients' strength of affiliation with American–Indian and white American cultural identities was examined. The results indicated that provider–patient differences were greater for patients affiliating weakly with white cultural identity than for those affiliating strongly.

> **SUMMARY**
>
> - Human beings have much in common, but our small or subtle differences define our uniqueness.
> - Cultural identity refers to the feeling of belonging to a group.
> - An understanding of cultural identity is essential for developing cultural competence.

Constructing 'otherness'

'Othering' may be viewed as a negative concept that focuses on difference in order to justify stigma, discrimination and marginalisation, unlike the concept of diversity, which represents positivity and a celebration of difference. According to Mengstie (2011), 'otherness' is a way of defining one's own 'self' or one's own 'identity' in relation to others. The term 'otherness' refers to being distinct or different from that which is otherwise experienced or known. The experience of being 'other' can be expressed in many ways, including age, ethnicity, sex, physical ability, sexual orientation, socio-economic class and other demographic factors. As with cultural identity, an understanding of the concept of otherness can also help us to develop cultural understanding, sensitivity and respect.

Most of us have at one time or another judged people in negative ways, simply because their behaviour, lifestyle and so on did not meet our own standards (Papadopoulos, 2006). However, sometimes we may assign identities to others based on physical characteristics and social constructs, which can be a harmful process if used to promote 'otherness' by pitting identity groups against one another or ascribing greater social value to particular identities (Sullivan, 2015).

According to Johnson, et al. (2009), 'othering' is a process that identifies those that are thought to be different from oneself or the mainstream, and it can reinforce and reproduce positions of domination and subordination. Utilising ethnographic methods involving interviews and focus group discussions, Johnson, et al. (2009) sought to explore the interactions between healthcare providers and South Asian immigrant women in order to describe othering practices. The process involved identifying uses of othering and exploring the dynamics through which this took place. Women shared stories of how discriminatory treatment was experienced, whilst the interviews with healthcare professionals provided examples of how the views of South Asian women shaped the way healthcare services were provided. Three forms of othering were identified in informants' descriptions of their problematic healthcare encounters: (a) essentialising explanations; (b) culturalist explanations; and (c) racialising explanations. The analysis demonstrated how individual interactions are influenced by the social and institutional contexts that create conditions for othering practices. These authors conclude that in order to foster safe and effective healthcare interactions, it is important to unmask othering practices and transform healthcare environments to support truly equitable healthcare (Johnson, et al., 2009).

A RECONSTRUCTED STORY OF 'OTHERING' BASED ON DATA FROM THE 'ENDOMETRIOSIS AND CULTURAL DIVERSITY' PROJECT

A Pakistani woman suffered with severe and prolonged menstrual period pain and painful sexual intercourse for almost seven years before she was diagnosed with endometriosis. She explained that her GP[2] dismissed her pain as normal and recommended she took pain killers. She opined that if she were a middle-class, assertive white woman, she would have been taken more seriously. She believed that the doctor had stereotyped her as an Asian woman who had a low pain threshold and a low sexual drive.

By essentialising the woman's health problems based on false assumptions and cultural stereotypes, the doctor was viewing the woman as different to the majority white population and was therefore committing an act of 'othering'. The doctor's 'othering' resulted in a dismissive attitude and lack of action, causing the woman unnecessary suffering for a long time. The doctor's behaviour may also be seen as discriminatory since the woman was denied the investigations and treatment that other women can access (Denny, et al., 2010).

Notions of otherness can easily lead to stigma, with which a number of health problems may be associated. Likewise, the concept of otherness may lead to discrimination. In a study aimed at investigating the effects of ethnic discrimination on the mental health of Ecuadorian immigrants in Spain and to assess the roles of material and social resources, ethnic discrimination was found to be associated with psychological distress in this immigrant population. These researchers suggest that discrimination effects may be exacerbated among those facing economic stress and those without economic support and that this particularly vulnerable group should be the subject of social and health interventions (Llacer, et al., 2009).

A further study by Nadimpalli, et al. (2016) explored the relationships between self-reported discrimination and mental and physical health among Sikh Asian Indians, suggesting that this group may be particularly discriminated against because of physical manifestations of their faith, including a tendency to wear turbans or ethnic clothing. These authors conclude that community-based efforts are needed to reduce or buffer the effects of discrimination experienced.

The UNESCO Universal Declaration on Cultural Diversity (2001, p.3) states that "each individual must acknowledge not only otherness in all its forms but also the plurality of his or her own identity, within societies that are themselves plural. Only in this way can cultural diversity be preserved as an adaptive process…"

Based on an analytical reading of Article II of the Universal Declaration on Bioethics and Human Rights (UNESCO, 2005), which states that no individual or group should be discriminated against or stigmatised on any grounds, in violation of human dignity, human rights and fundamental freedoms, and taking universal human rights as a reference, Godoi and Garrafa (2014) propose the consideration of the key concepts of identity, otherness, difference and tolerance in order to better understand the processes of producing stigma and discrimination. These authors suggest that it is from the experience of otherness – of looking at the other and being looked at – that we can look at and perceive ourselves. Stigma and discrimination represent the opposites of recognising otherness – they are the denial of tolerance in the sense of respecting difference (Godoi and Garrafa, 2014).

However, as discussed in the earlier sections of this chapter, the experience of otherness may not represent the main influencing factor on how we perceive ourselves, as the values that derive from our families and cultural groups are also strongly influential. But the concept of 'otherness' may be central to understanding how majority and minority identities are constructed, and therefore an understanding of 'otherness' may be crucial in the development of cultural knowledge and sensitivity.

SUMMARY

- Otherness represents a way of defining one's self or one's own identity in relation to others.
- Othering is a process that identifies those that are thought to be different from oneself.
- The concept of otherness may lead to stigma, with which a number of health problems may be associated.
- Othering may be viewed as a negative concept that focuses on difference in order to justify stigma, discrimination and marginalisation.
- As with cultural identity, an understanding of the concept of otherness can also help us to develop cultural understanding, sensitivity and respect.
- The concept of 'otherness' may be central to understanding how majority and minority identities are constructed, and therefore an understanding of 'otherness' may be crucial in the development of cultural competence.

Socio-cultural determinants of health

Understanding socio-cultural determinants of health is of great importance in enhancing cultural competence in healthcare, recognising and challenging discrimination and achieving health equity. As discussed earlier, health is determined by several factors, including culture, genetic inheritance, personal behaviours, access to quality healthcare and the general external environment (Hernandez and Blazer, 2006). As reported by the Centers for Disease Control and Prevention (n.d.), health equity represents an opportunity for everyone to attain their full health potential whereby no one is disadvantaged from achieving this potential because of their social position or other socially determined circumstance. Furthermore, health equity may be defined as the absence of systematic disparities in health between and within social groups who exhibit different levels of underlying social advantages or disadvantages. It is suggested that socio-cultural determinants of health such as poverty, unequal access to healthcare, lack of education, stigma and racism are underlying, contributing factors of health inequities. Thus, health organisations, institutions and education programmes are encouraged to look beyond behavioural and biological factors and to address underlying factors related to socio-cultural determinants of health (Centers for Disease Control and Prevention, n.d.).

The same message is also given by the World Health Organization (WHO; www.who.int/hia/evidence/doh/en), which reminds us that many factors combine together to affect the health of individuals and communities. Whether people are healthy or not is determined by their circumstances and environment. The WHO suggest that key determinants of health include:

- The social and economic environment
- The physical environment
- The person's individual characteristics and behaviours

The Public Health Agency of Canada also assert that age, sex and heredity are key factors that determine health (www.canada.ca/en/public-health/services/health-promotion/population-health/what-determines-health.html).

The choices we make also matter, but these choices are influenced by environments, experiences, cultures and other factors. Socio-cultural determinants strongly interact to influence health, and improvement in any of these may produce improvement in both health behaviours and outcomes among individuals and groups.

In this chapter, evidence has been presented to support the view that not only social but also cultural determinants of health must be considered as important factors to our health. Over time, health has been defined in different ways. Health is one of the most important humanistic values and it is a prerequisite for the realisation of all other values. Moreover, health is a determinant of the ability to satisfactorily perform socio-cultural tasks and roles, as well as to gain achievements of a socio-economic nature. Individual responsibility for health is to a large extent based on the belief that health is not only a human right, but also an investment, the consequence of which is the ability to have the choice of specific services and health behaviours (Stawarz, et al., 2014).

SUMMARY

- Health is determined by a number of factors, including culture, personal behaviours, access to quality healthcare and the general environment.
- Whether people are healthy or not may be determined by their circumstances and environment.
- It is suggested that social determinants of health such as poverty, unequal access to healthcare, lack of education, stigma and racism are underlying, contributing factors of health inequities.
- Social and cultural determinants of health must be considered as equally important factors.
- Socio-cultural determinants strongly interact to influence health.
- Health is a determinant of the ability to satisfactorily perform socio-cultural tasks.

Cultural competence

The previous sections of this chapter demonstrated the need for health professionals who can design, develop and deliver culturally competent services. Ten years ago, I defined cultural competence as "the capacity to provide effective healthcare taking into consideration people's cultural beliefs, behaviours and needs" (Papadopoulos, 2006, p.11).

We all use the term 'effective' to encompass many things, such as appropriate, acceptable, compassionate, giving the desired results and so on. All these messages are hidden in this all-encompassing term. So, in my Anna Reynvaan Lecture of 2011, I redefined cultural competence as "the capacity to provide effective and compassionate healthcare taking into consideration people's cultural beliefs, behaviours and needs."

Cultural competence is both a process and an output and it results from the synthesis of the knowledge and skills that we acquire during our personal and professional lives. A culturally competent health professional is one who possesses the virtue of courage to challenge accepted norms and practices that harm, discriminate or disadvantage the users of the healthcare services.

The case of Mrs Hassan

Let us consider the case of a seventy-year-old Turkish woman, Mrs Hassan, who arrived from Turkey five years ago to stay with her only son who has been living in England with his wife and two children for the last fifteen years. Mrs Hassan does not speak English. Just over a year ago, she noticed a lump on her breast but did not say anything to her son or daughter-in-law as she was embarrassed and also she did not want to bother them. They both worked full time and often left home early in the morning and came back late and very tired. Being a faithful Muslim, Mrs Hassan believed that Allah can heal diseases so she read the Koran and prayed five times a day. Recently, her family noticed that she was losing weight and she often complained of aches and pains. She is now in hospital and has been diagnosed with advanced-stage breast cancer and secondary deposits in her lungs.

The team who is looking after Mrs Hassan includes an English, a Spanish and a Nigerian nurse (all female), an English male consultant, a Bulgarian female junior doctor and a female Filipino healthcare assistant.

Mrs Hassan's son informed the nurses that he does not wish them to tell his mother about her diagnosis. He wants to protect and spare his mother from all the distress she would have if she knew her diagnosis. He also wishes his mother to be given all available treatments in order to arrest the cancer and give her the best chances for life. He does not see the need for a professional interpreter as he has taken time off work in order that he and his wife and teenage children can be available to act as translators.

What are some of the challenges for Mrs Hassan and the caring team?

- She has not been in England long enough to acculturate and she probably spent most of her time at home looking after the family.
- As a result, she does not speak English; further, she is not adequately familiar with the healthcare system.
- Her age, religious background and collectivist cultural identity may mean that she will comply with the decisions made on her behalf by her family and the healthcare team.
- She will wonder if the healthcare team understand her cultural/religious rituals and traditions that she would like to observe.

- She is frightened being in a strange environment and unable to communicate on her own.
- She worries that the staff will not like her because she is a foreigner and different from them and wonders whether they will ignore her because she cannot communicate with them.

However, there are challenges within the healthcare team as well. The members of the team have different religious and cultural backgrounds. Some were born and grew up in England, others have been living in the country for a number of years, whilst others have only recently moved to England having grown up and been educated in a different country. In addition, half of the members have only recently joined the team. All of these factors can influence the dynamics of the team and may impact on the care of Mrs Hassan. Their differences in cultural and religious values, their understanding of professional hierarchies and gender differences and their own educational, professional and life experiences can be barriers to effective communication.

The case of Mrs Hasan is by no means unique to England; similar cases are repeated the world over. Sensitive, appropriate, acceptable, compassionate care is an undisputed human right in the professional codes of all caring professions that are firmly built on human rights. The ethics that underpin human rights are extensively connected to the Aristotelian virtue ethics that are evident in this book.

The PTT model of cultural competence

Let us examine some of the challenges facing the team caring for Mrs Hassan using the notions of the PTT model of transcultural health and cultural competence (see Figure 4.1) (Papadopoulos, 2006).

As you can see, the model consists of four main constructs: (a) cultural awareness; (b) cultural knowledge; (c) cultural sensitivity; and (d) cultural competence. A conceptual map is provided for each stage as a guideline only. Educators may add other concepts or modify the proposed ones to suit their type and level of students.

(a) Cultural awareness

The first stage in the model is cultural awareness, which begins with an examination of our personal values and beliefs. So, how does the notion of cultural awareness help to provide culturally competent care for Mrs Hassan?

Spending a little time thinking about our own cultural background will make us realise what values we hold and why. Hopefully, we will discover values, attitudes and beliefs that are hidden deep in our subconscious but could surface when we are stressed, demonstrating that, like all human beings, we too can stereotype and be ethnocentric. But this self-reflection will help us prepare for when such events happen.

Spending time to find out some information related to Mrs Hassan's cultural identity and ethnohistory, such as where she comes from, why she left her country and what values she holds, will make us realise that even though all human beings have much in common, our small or subtle differences are important, as they are the ones that define our uniqueness and our individuality.

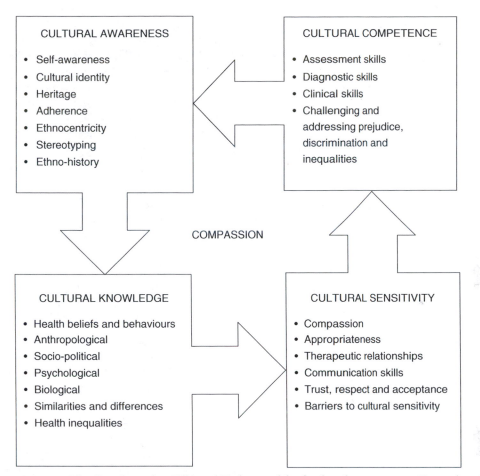

FIGURE 4.1 The Papadopoulos, Tilki and Taylor model of cultural competence. Reproduced with permission.

Source: This figure was published in Transcultural health and social care. Development of culturally competent practitioners, 2006, Elsevier.

An obvious difference between Mrs Hassan and the nurses is likely to be religion. As an older woman, she may still hold the view that as a patient she must listen unquestionably and do what the doctors and nurses tell her to do. As a Muslim, she will want to pray several times a day and will believe that Allah may give health problems to people but also can take them away. She will most likely accept her son's judgements and will rely on his guidance as someone who understands both the language and the healthcare systems. Some members of the healthcare team may find her behaviour to be passive, something that is often considered negative by healthcare staff who have been socialised to believe that it is best for individuals to be actively involved in their care. Not being able to communicate directly with her makes it harder for them to know what she really thinks and wants or to question the stereotypes they hold about her.

(b) Cultural knowledge

The next major construct of the model is cultural knowledge, which can be gained in a number of ways, such as meaningful contact with ordinary people from different ethnic groups in the societies we live or during travelling to other countries, as well as from knowledge produced by disciplines such as anthropology, sociology, psychology and others. All of these sources can enhance our knowledge of the health beliefs and behaviours of people whose cultures differ from our own, as well as raise our understanding around the problems they face.

Learning from our patients is another way to gain cultural knowledge. This is based on the belief that a person's culture is individually and socially constructed and reconstructed rather than being a static entity. Individual differences exist within any culture and this should be acknowledged by healthcare professionals through questioning and verification. However, this approach is not always possible, such as when a patient is unconscious or extremely ill or when a patient cannot speak the language, like Mrs Hassan. Therefore, having some culture-generic knowledge, which can be gained during training, is an essential preparation and a good starting point for such occasions, until the interpreters are in place or family members are available. Caution should be exercised in the use of both family members and/or professional interpreters as there are both practical and ethical advantages and disadvantages to using them.

Health inequalities are given serious attention within the PTT model. This is because even though all human beings are cultural beings and therefore their cultural beliefs and behaviours should be taken into consideration, we know that health inequalities in developed countries are far more extensive in people from minority ethnic groups as compared with indigenous majority populations. It would be convenient to blame the health inequalities experienced by these people on their culture, as some politicians and even health professionals try to do. But the evidence that has amassed over the last thirty years points to the fact that these health inequalities are linked to structural inequalities and discrimination experienced by people from minority ethnic groups, such as poor housing, unemployment, lack of educational opportunities, social exclusion and inaccessible health services (Stevenson, 2014; Evandrou, et al., 2016).

How have cultural and structural determinants resulted in health inequality for Mrs Hassan? Coming from a highly collective culture, Mrs Hassan most probably saw her role as the family carer. Arriving in England at the age of sixty-five, she felt strong and able to devote all of her time to activities that made the life of her busy son and his wife a little easier. However, spending most of her time at home left very little time for her to do anything else, such as attending English language classes. But there may also be structural reasons for her inability to learn English, such as the unavailability of English courses in the area of her residence or the availability of them at times that are inconvenient to her. Not being able to communicate with the world outside her home meant that Mrs Hassan would not have been confident enough to make an appointment to see her GP when she discovered the lump on her breast, something that would have given her a more positive outcome and a better chance for life.

(c) Cultural sensitivity

An important element in achieving cultural sensitivity is how professionals view those in their care. Cultural sensitivity requires equal patient–health professional partnerships involving compassion, trust, acceptance and respect, as well as facilitation and negotiation. A key factor of cultural sensitivity is learning to ask the right questions. Having the necessary awareness and culture-generic knowledge will enable the nurse or other health professionals to anticipate needs and ask questions with the right content and in the right manner, thus minimising the risk of communication barriers and misunderstandings. Although Mrs Hassan's son and his family are prepared to interpret for her, the healthcare team needs to ensure that this is what Mrs Hassan wants. This should be done on admission or soon after. She may express the wish to discuss certain issues with someone outside the family, such as a professional interpreter. It is also necessary for the healthcare team to assess on admission Mrs Hassan's understanding of her health problem without the presence of her son or other members of the family. It is essential to ask such questions as:

- What do you *call* your problem?
- What do you think *caused* your problem?
- How do you *cope* with your condition?
- What *concerns* do you have regarding your condition?

(Slavin, Kuo and Galanti, n.d.)

Her answers to these questions will provide many cultural clues that will enable the nurse and her colleagues to establish a therapeutic relationship with Mrs Hassan based on respect for her culture, concern about her dignity – especially in relation to the gender of the healthcare professionals engaging in physical assessments or other interventions – and a compassionate approach that communicates to her that the healthcare team recognises her needs, pain and anxiety and are there to help, support and care for her.

Regular use of an interpreter to explain her care every step of the way and encourage her to ask questions, responding to any requests that she may make and accepting her ways of eating, washing and praying without making her feel embarrassed and strange are all appropriate actions. Above all, nurses need to recognise that her family are very important to her and so should allow her to see them without too many restrictions of time and numbers of visitors.

Involving her family in her care and decision-making is also important. She will expect this. Finding a way to negotiate the differences between her son's views and the healthcare team's views is another priority that must be handled sensitively. The healthcare team must try to understand why her son feels the way he does and explain their reasons for having different views. Patients and family members also have stereotypes about health professionals and the health services. They have probably heard stories from their friends who may have had negative experiences and so fear this may happen to them. They may have suspicions about things that they do not understand and have not had explained. However, with sensitivity and patience, most people find solutions and reach compromises.

(d) Cultural competence

The achievement of cultural competence requires the synthesis and application of previously gained awareness, knowledge and sensitivity in the practice of assessing the patient's needs, her clinical diagnosis and the caring interventions. A most important component of this stage is the ability to recognise and challenge racism and other forms of discrimination and oppressive practice.

However, the act of challenging requires courage. Aristotle taught that courage without wisdom is dangerous for both the person who is committing the unwise courageous act and the persons to whom this is committed. Gaining the wisdom to recognise unfairness and to challenge it effectively is a virtue we must learn in similar ways as those we have discussed in other sections and chapters of this book that relate to compassion (see Chapters 5 and 6).

We have considered in the section 'Cultural sensitivity' the use of the four C questions developed by Slavin, Kuo and Galanti (n.d.) as one way of assessing the patient's problem. Another good way to assess and plan culturally competent care for Mrs Hassan is by following the LEARN principles as proposed by Berlin and Fowkes in 1982.

The LEARN model stands for:

L – 'Listen' to her perception of her problem.
E – 'Explain' your perception of the problem.
A – 'Acknowledge' the similarities and differences between the two.
R – 'Recommend' with her involvement and that of her family.
N – 'Negotiate' the treatment plan, which incorporates relevant aspects of Mrs Hassan's culture, as well as her and her family's wishes.

Concluding remarks

It is of great importance to realise that different cultural and ethnic groups may differ in terms of their values, beliefs and behaviours. Within this chapter, a number of key concepts have been discussed aimed at contributing to our understanding of health and illness in multicultural societies, thus enhancing our ability to deliver care that is culturally competent and compassionate. Working in healthcare settings within multicultural societies involves interacting with people from a number of different cultural backgrounds and it is important for nurses to understand their own values and beliefs so that they can better understand those of their patients.

An understanding of personal values and cultural identities can help us to develop cultural awareness, sensitivity and respect, as can an understanding of the concept of 'otherness'. Otherness may represent one way of defining one's own 'self', but it can also be viewed as a negative concept that focuses on difference in order to justify stigma, discrimination and marginalisation.

It is suggested that socio-cultural determinants of health, such as poverty, level of education, ethnicity, cultural background, stigma and racism, can all contribute to health inequities. Understanding such factors may enhance cultural competence and aid in the recognition of discrimination and the achievement of health equity, resulting in better health and the alleviation of illness.

All the above concepts and factors were taken into consideration when developing the PTT model of cultural competence, the key elements of which were applied to the case of Mrs Hassan in order to exemplify its usefulness and simplicity.

Culturally competent and compassionate care is excellent care and this should be afforded to all peoples. As health professionals, we should always endeavour to do the right thing for the right reasons. Aristotle taught us that:

> Excellence is an art won by training and habituation. We do not act rightly because we have virtue or excellence, but we rather have those because we have acted rightly. We are what we repeatedly do. Excellence, then, is not an act but a habit.
>
> *(Attributed to Aristotle)*

LEARNING ACTIVITIES

- Write some notes on how you think an understanding of personal values, cultural identities, otherness and socio-cultural determinants of health may enhance your efforts to provide culturally competent and compassionate healthcare.
- Write a couple of sentences on your own beliefs and personal values.
- Explain the extent to which you feel your own personal beliefs influence your approach towards others.
- Read the poem *We and They* by Rudyard Kipling (www.wales.nhs.uk/sitesplus/documents/829/Rudyard%20Kipling.pdf). Reflect on the poem for a few minutes and then write down your reflections by responding to the following questions:
  - What was the main topic of the poem?
  - Why, in your view, did the poet feel the need to write this poem?
  - What is the main message of the poem?
- What are your thoughts about the PTT model of cultural competence?
- Is this a model that you could adopt in your practice (nursing, medicine, other healthcare occupations, teaching or researching)?
- If you had to talk about the model to a group of colleagues, what would you say and how would you explain its main constructs?

Notes

1 The author acknowledges the help of Sue Shea in the preparation of this chapter.
2 A general practitioner is a primary health doctor; people with a health problem must consult him/her in the first instance. Referring the person to a specialist doctor is at his/her decision.

References

Adler, P. (2002). Beyond cultural identity: Reflections on multiculturalism. Retrieved from www.mediate.com/articles/adler3.cfm.

American College of Obstetricians and Gynecologists (2011). ACOG *Committee Opinion No. 493*: Cultural sensitivity and awareness in the delivery of health care. *Obstetrics and Gynecology*, 117, pp. 1258–1261.

Berlin, E. and Fowkes, W. (1982). A teaching framework for cross-cultural health care. *Western Journal of Medicine*, 139 (6), pp. 934–938.

Campbell, R.D. and Long, L.A. (2014). Culture as a social determinant of mental and behavioural health: A look at culturally shaped beliefs and their impact on help-seeking behaviours and service use patterns of black Americans with depression. *Best Practices in Mental Health*, 10(2), pp. 48–62.

Centers for Disease Control and Prevention (n.d.). Retrieved September 2016 from: www.cdc.gov/nchhstp/socialdeterminants/faq.html.

Clapton, J. and Fitzgerald, J. (n.d.). The history of disability: a history of 'otherness' how disable people have been marginalized through the ages and their present struggle for their human rights. Retrieved from: www.ru.org/index.php/human-rights/315-the-history-of-disability-a-history-of-otherness.

Denny, E., Culley, L., Papadopoulos, I. and Apenteng, P. (2010). Endometriosis and cultural diversity: Improving services for minority ethnic women. *Final report for Research for Patient Benefit grant PB-PG-0906-11145*. Birmingham, UK, Birmingham City University.

Evandrou, M., Falkingham, J., Feng, Z. and Vlachantoni, A. (2016). Ethnic inequalities in limiting health and self-reported health in later life revisited. *Journal of Epidemiology and Community Health*, 70(7), pp. 653–662.

Garroutte, E.M., Sarkisian, N., Aeguelles, L., Goldberg, J. and Buchwald, D. (2006). Cultural identities and perceptions of health among health care providers and older American Indians. *Journal of General Internal Medicine*, 21(2), pp. 111–116.

General Medical Council (2013). How could a patient's personal beliefs affect their healthcare? Retrieved from: www.gmc-uk.org/guidance/ethical_guidance/21179.asp.

Godoi, A.M.M. and Garrafa, V. (2014). Bioethics reading of the principle of non-discrimination and non-stigmatization. *Saúde e Sociedade*, 23(1), p.110.

Groen, S. (2009). Recognizing cultural identity in mental health care: Rethinking the cultural formulation of a Somali patient. *Transcultural Psychiatry*, 46(3), pp. 451–462.

Hack, S.M., Larrison, C.R. and Gone, J.P. (2014). American Indian identity in mental health services utilization data from a rural Midwestern sample. *Cultural Diversity and Ethnic Minority Psychology*, 20(1), pp. 68–74.

Hernandez, L.M. and Blazer, D.G., eds. (2006). *Genes, behavior, and the social environment: Moving beyond the nature/nurture debate*. Washington, DC, USA, National Academies Press.

Johnson, J.L., Bottorff, J.L., Browne, A.J., Grewal, S., Hilton, B.A. and Clarke, H. (2009). Othering and being othered in the context of health care services. *Health Communication*, 16(2), pp. 253–271.

Kung, F.Y.H., Eibach, R.P. and Grossmann, I. (2016). Culture, fixed-world beliefs, relationships, and perceptions of identity change. *Social Psychological and Personality Science*, 7(7), pp. 631–639.

Lang, T., Lepage, B., Schieber, A.C., Lamy, S. and Kelly-Irving, M. (2012). Social determinants of cardiovascular diseases. *Public Health Reviews*, 33, pp. 601–622.

Leininger, M.M. (1991). *Culture care diversity and universality. A theory of nursing*. New York, NY: NLN.

Llácer, A., Del Amo, J., García-Fulgueiras, A., Ibáñez-Rojo, V., García-Pino, R., Jarrín, I., Díaz, D., Fernández-Liria, A, … Zunzunegui, M.V. (2009). Discrimination and mental health in Ecuadorian immigrants in Spain. *Journal of Epidemiology and Community Health*, 63, pp. 766–772.

Mc Laughlin, L. and Braun, K. (1998). Asian and Pacific Islander cultural values: Considerations for health care decision-making. *Health and Social Work*, 23(2), pp. 116–126.

Mengstie, S. (2011). Constructions of 'otherness' and the role of education: The case of Ethiopia. *Journal of Education Culture and Society*, 2, pp. 7–15.

Nadimpalli, S.B., Cleland, C.M., Hutchinson, M.K., Islam, N., Barnes, L.L. and Van Devanter, N. (2016). The association between discrimination and the health of Sikh Asian Indians. *Health Psychology*, 35(4), pp. 351–355.

Owuor, J.O.A. and Nake, J.N. (2015) *Internalised stigma as a barrier to access to health and social care services by minority ethnic groups in the UK*. London, UK: Race Equality Foundation.

Oxford, J. (2012). Relating your values, morals and ethics to nursing practice. *Independent Nurse*. Retrieved from: www.independentnurse.co.uk/professional-article/relating-your-values-morals-and-ethics-to-nursing-practice/64200.

Papadopoulos, I., ed. (2006). *Transcultural health and social care: Development of culturally competent practitioners.* Edinburgh, UK: Churchill Livingstone Elsevier.

Public Health Agency of Canada (n.d.). Social and economic factors that influence our health and contribute to health inequalities. Retrieved January 2018 from: www.canada.ca/en/public-health/corporate/publications/chief-public-health-officer-reports-state-public-health-canada/report-on-state-public-health-canada-2008/chapter-4a.html.

Rassin, M. (2008). Nurses' professional and personal values. *Nursing Ethics*, 15(5), pp. 614–630.

Simonds, V.W., Goins, R.T., Krantz, E.M. and Garroutte, E.M. (2014). Cultural identity and patient trust among older American Indians. *Journal of General Internal Medicine*, 29(3), pp. 500–506.

Slavin, S., Galanti, G.A. and Kuo, A. (n.d.). The 4 C's of culture: A mnemonic for health care professionals. Retrieved January 2018 from: www.ggalanti.org/the-4cs-of-culture.

Stawarz, B., Sulima, M., Lewicka, M., Brukwicka, I. and Wiktor, H. (2014). Health and determinants of health – A review of literature. *Journal of Public Health, Nursing and Medical Rescue*, 2, pp. 4–10.

Stevenson, J. (2014). *Explaining levels of wellbeing in BME populations in England.* London, UK: Institute of Health and Human Development, University of East London.

Sullivan, K. (2015). *Otherness and the power of exclusion.* Sockholm International Peace Research Institute. Retrieved from: www.sipri.org/commentary/blog/2015/otherness-and-power-exclusion.

Tanyas, B. (2016). Experiences of otherness and practices of othering: Young Turkish migrants in the UK. *Young*, 24(2), pp. 157–173.

UNESCO Universal Declaration on Cultural Diversity (2001). Retrieved from: www.unesco.org/fileadmin/MULTIMEDIA/HQ/CLT/pdf/5_Cultural_Diversity_EN.pdf.

UNESCO (2005). *Universal declaration on bioethics and human rights.* Paris, France: UNESCO.

5

THE PAPADOPOULOS MODEL OF CULTURALLY COMPETENT COMPASSION

LEARNING OBJECTIVES

Upon completion of this chapter, readers should be able to:

- Defining culturally competent compassion.
- Outline the origins of the Papadopoulos conceptual model for culturally competent compassion.
- List the building blocks of the model.
- Describe the four constructs of the model.
- Appreciate the significance of the first massive open online course on culturally competent compassion in healthcare.
- Outline the results of the first international survey on culturally competent compassion in healthcare.

Introduction

In the previous three chapters, we examined how compassion is defined, understood and practised by some of the major religions and have discussed the views of a number of influential philosophers who lived during the last 2500 years. We discovered the near-universal agreement that compassion is an emotion that leads human beings to acts of 'self' and 'other' comfort and alleviation of suffering. We also discovered that, in addition to a high level of universal agreement on the benefits of compassion, the various religions and philosophers interpret specific elements and actions associated with compassion in different ways. These differences may be viewed as the result of variations in time and place, as well as other factors and events that shape values and beliefs. All such phenomena may be viewed as culture. Hall and Jefferson (1996, pp. 10–11) defined culture as:

The culture of a group or class is the peculiar and distinctive 'way of life' of the group, the meanings, values and ideas embodied in institutions, in systems of belief, in mores and customs, in the uses of objects and material life. Culture is the distinctive shape in which this material and social organisation of life expresses itself. A culture includes the 'maps of meaning' which make things intelligible to its members. …Culture is the way the social relations of a group are structured and shaped: but it is also the way those shapes are experienced, understood and interpreted.

Figure 5.1 provides a summary of some of the key elements of culture that can impact on the meaning and interpretation of compassion.

Based on this indivisible understanding of culture and compassion, it is curious why the vast literature on compassion treats compassion as though it has no connection to culture – in other words, as an acultural concept. The one exception is by Goetz, et al. (2010), who assert that the ways in which compassion functions – the reduction of suffering and the formation and maintenance of cooperative relationships – almost certainly vary across cultures. They hypothesised the possibility that cultures that are very interdependent (collectivist) may have a tendency to feel compassion for in-group members, while independent cultures (individual-istic) may have a tendency to feel compassion for out-group members. However, this hypoth-esis remains unproven. As a general rule, cultures vary in their outward displays of emotion, thus we can conclude that this rule also applies to compassion.

This chapter introduces you to the Papadopoulos model of culturally competent compas-sion (Figure 5.2). As has been discussed in earlier chapters of this book, nursing, particularly in the UK, has been putting the spotlight on compassion in recent years and, as a result, several

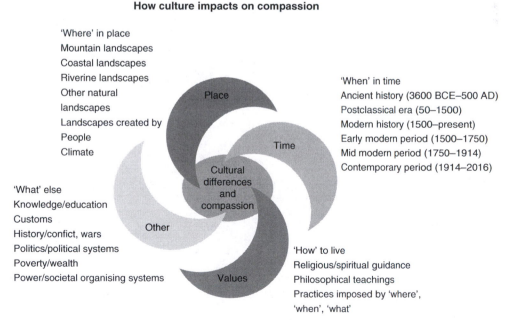

How culture impacts on compassion

'Where' in place
Mountain landscapes
Coastal landscapes
Riverine landscapes
Other natural
landscapes
Landscapes created by
People
Climate

Place

Time

'When' in time
Ancient history (3600 BCE–500 AD)
Postclassical era (50–1500)
Modern history (1500–present)
Early modern period (1500–1750)
Mid modern period (1750–1914)
Contemporary period (1914–2016)

Cultural
differences
and
compassion

'What' else
Knowledge/education
Customs
History/confict, wars
Politics/political systems
Poverty/wealth
Power/societal organising systems

Other

Values

'How' to live
Religious/spiritual guidance
Philosophical teachings
Practices imposed by 'where',
'when', 'what'

FIGURE 5.1 How culture impacts on compassion.

practice, research and policy initiatives have been developed and implemented and numerous scholarly works have been published (Chambers and Ryder, 2009; Francis, 2010; Sellman, 2011; Cummings and Bennett, 2012; Baughan and Smith, 2013; Shea, et al., 2014; Hewison and Sawbridge, 2016).

In 2009, the King's Fund published the report *The point of care. Enabling compassionate care in acute hospital settings* (Firth-Cozens and Cornwell, 2009). In it, the authors discuss some of the definitions that were used at the time. They found that compassion was often conflated with the notions of empathy, respect, recognition of the uniqueness of another individual and willingness to enter into a relationship in which not only the knowledge but the intuitions, strengths and emotions of both the patient and the physician can be fully engaged (Lowenstein, 2008). They also reported the simpler definition used by Chochinov (2007) of compassion as a deep awareness of the suffering of another coupled with the wish to relieve it. They reminded us that when the UK's NHS Constitution (Department of Health, 2009) discusses compassion, it states:

> We respond with humanity and kindness to each person's pain, distress, anxiety or need. We search for the things we can do, however small, to give comfort and relieve suffering. We find time for those we serve and work alongside. We do not wait to be asked, because we care.

For Frank (2004), compassion – both giving and receiving it – entails an emotional response. It goes beyond acts of basic care and is likely to involve generosity (giving a little more than you have to), kindness and real dialogue.

Firth-Cozens and Cornwell (2009, p.3) go on to explain:

> ...real dialogue is a vital part of compassion and of good care in general. It is more than communication, which is the accurate giving and receiving of a message. It is spoken human to human rather than clinician to patient; it shows interest; never stereotypes but recognises and enjoys difference while also appreciating the common core of humanity; it includes honesty where necessary, and may need courage at times. This form of dialogue is crucial if the patient is to be seen as a whole person and should be engaged in by staff at all points of health care.

van der Cingel (2011) conducted qualitative research and analysed in-depth interviews with nurses and patients in order to answer the question: 'What is the nature and significance of compassion for older people with a chronic disease in nursing practice?' The research involved interviews with thirty nurses and thirty-one patients with a variety of chronic diseases in The Netherlands. The analysis yielded the following seven dimensions of compassion:

1. Attentiveness
2. Listening
3. Confronting: verbalisation of suffering – acknowledging and valuing by the nurse
4. Involvement
5. Helping: assisting with activities of daily living that the patient can no longer perform
6. Presence: being there
7. Understanding.

Strauss, et al. (2016), in search of an elusive consensus on a definition of compassion that they suggest is necessary for scientific enquiry into compassion and the development of robust measuring tools, conducted an extensive review of the literature, which led them to identify the following five components of compassion that can be found in most definitions:

1. Recognition of suffering
2. Understanding its universality
3. Feeling sympathy, empathy or concern for those who are suffering
4. Tolerating the distress associated with the witnessing of suffering
5. Motivation to act or acting to alleviate suffering.

My journey to culturally competent and compassionate nursing education

I started researching transcultural nursing education in the late 1980s. In 1998, I published with two colleagues the Papadopoulos, Tilki and Taylor (PTT) model of transcultural nursing and cultural competence, which I further developed in 2006 (Papadopoulos, et al., 1998; Papadopoulos, 2006). In 2008, I embarked on the Intercultural Education for Nurses in Europe (IENE) programme, which is currently on its seventh project (www. ieneproject.eu). The initial motivation for the establishment of the programme was to help nurses' mobility within the European Union; thus, the aim was compatible with the vision of education for world citizenship. Whilst the first and second IENE projects focused totally on aspects of intercultural nursing education, the third and subsequent projects have and are addressing aspects of intercultural compassion in health and nursing education.

I became interested in compassion in 2010 when I became a grandmother for the first time. During the immediate period before and after the birth of my grandchild, I observed and experienced first-hand culturally insensitive care that was void of compassion. Shortly after, the Francis report (2010) into the Mid Staffordshire hospital scandal was published. These two critical incidents provided the stimulus to review my thinking around my definition of cultural competence. I had assumed that compassion was a coherent part of cultural competence that did not need to be spelled out. I had taken for granted the essence of nursing care (compassion), as others had done before me, the result of which was to silence what we all considered obvious and therefore did not need to be explained. Compassion was assumed to be such an inseparable part of everything we taught, learnt and practised that it did not need to be theorized on or taught as a separate entity.

Following the publication of the Francis report, the debate about compassion took off. The mass media, social media and professional journals all featured items on compassion. Researchers, policy-makers and professional bodies produced articles, policy reports and strategies for practice and education. Unfortunately, all of these publications referred to compassion in universal terms. None of them discussed, investigated or acknowledged the possibility that, even though compassion may be a universal notion, it may nevertheless be understood and enacted in different ways by different cultures. This is the kind of compassion I am interested in. Combining my work on intercultural education, which includes cultural competence, and my curiosity about compassion resulted in the notion that I coined in 2011 as 'culturally competent compassion'. My working definition of it is:

> Culturally competent compassion is the human quality of understanding the suffering of others and wanting to do something about it, using culturally appropriate and acceptable interventions, which take into consideration both the patients' and the carers' cultural backgrounds as well as the context in which care is given.
>
> *(Papadopoulos, 2011)*

A model for culturally competent and compassionate praxis

In 2014, I published my conceptual model for developing culturally competent and compassionate health professionals (Figure 5.2). The notion of praxis is used here to mean the symbiosis of theory and practice. Using the concept of competence is compatible with the notion of praxis because competence is a term that encompasses knowledge, skills and attitudes.

The model was based on the following building blocks: (a) values, (b) principles and (c) the PTT framework (Figure 5.3).

As can be seen from Figure 5.2, key constructs relating to compassion have been overlaid on top of the original PTT model (see Chapter 4) constructs for cultural competence: (1) cultural awareness (which in the new model becomes cultural awareness and compassion); (2) cultural knowledge (which becomes cultural knowledge and compassion); (3) cultural sensitivity (which becomes cultural sensitivity and compassion); and (4) cultural competence (which becomes cultural competence and compassion). The familiar structure of the four key constructs provides the logical steps and the basic content map for the development of a systematic learning plan that can be embedded in any curriculum. The underpinning values of the model are derived from human rights and the notions of world citizenship. The educational principles informing the model are those of intercultural education (Huber, 2012; see Chapter 6).

Human rights have been a pillar of the PTT model for transcultural nursing and the development of culturally competent health workers since its inception in 1998. This was clearly articulated by Tilki (2006), who stated that human rights are the essence of transcultural care, and it is the right of every human being to be treated with dignity and respect and to have access to effective healthcare. The United Nations Declaration of Universal Human Rights and the European Convention on Human Rights promote, amongst others, equality, freedom from discrimination, freedom from degrading treatment, freedom of belief and religion, the right to participate in the cultural life of the community and so on. These declarations are based on the belief that all human beings are born free and equal in dignity and rights and that they are endowed with reason and conscience and should act towards one another in a spirit of brotherhood (Universal Declaration of Human Rights – United Nations, 1948). With increasing levels of globalisation and global migration, it is incumbent upon nurses and other health professionals to provide culturally competent and compassionate care to 'world citizens', thus contributing towards the creation of a healthier and more equal world. The principles of intercultural education reinforce the underpinning values of the model. The International Commission on Education for the Twenty-first Century (Delors, 1996) launched the project 'Learning to Live Together' (UNESCO, 2014). The project's vision was that in a highly

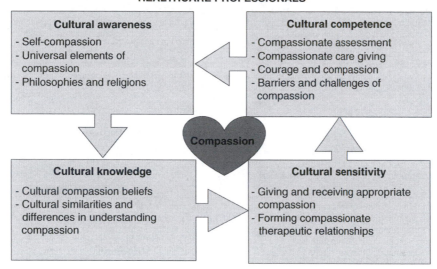

FIGURE 5.2 The Papadopoulos model for developing culturally competent and compassionate healthcare professionals.

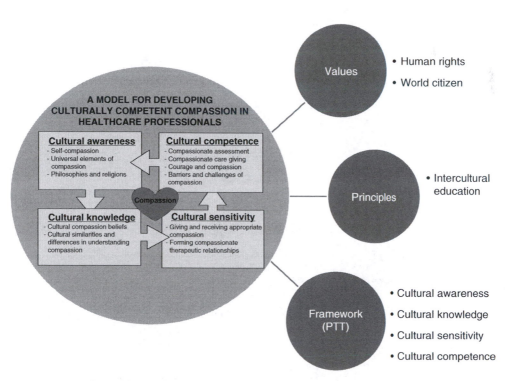

FIGURE 5.3 The model's building blocks.

globalised society, individuals, groups and communities should refer to human rights as the basis of living together. It emphasises the value of intercultural education due to its potential for cross-fertilisation, equality of cultures, multiple identities, acceptance of diversity and cooperative learning. It is therefore clear to see that the underpinning values and principles of the Papadopoulos model for developing culturally competent compassion in healthcare professionals embraces wider and non-traditional aspects of knowledge and skills necessary for the development and delivery of quality, culturally competent and compassionate services for all people.

The four constructs of the Papadopoulos model for developing culturally competent compassion in healthcare

(a) Cultural awareness and compassion

As discussed in Chapter 4, the starting point of the lifelong process of achieving culturally competent compassion is an awareness of our own cultural values and identities and the need for self- compassion. This is augmented by a critical consideration of the universal aspects of compassion, as well as how philosophers and religions have dealt with compassion over the years (see Chapters 2 and 3). Self- compassion is based on the Socratic dictum of 'know thyself'. 'Know thyself' (aftognosia) is the path to a virtuous life; this guides our actions towards understanding, caring and respecting our self. As our self is not complete without a relationship with another self, the virtue of compassion (symponia) provides the understanding of suffering of the other, whilst self-compassion, according to Neff (2011), involves not only understanding of our self, but treating it with kindness, caring and concern (see Box 5.1).

(b) Cultural knowledge and compassion

The second construct of the model consists of both a critical examination of how cultural beliefs inform our notion of compassion and a reflection on how our cultural similarities and differences relate to and impact on compassion.

BOX 5.1 CULTURAL AWARENESS AND COMPASSION REFLECTION ACTIVITY

Some relevant questions to reflect on are:

- Am I aware of my own worldview and what influenced and shaped it?
- How do my cultural values impact on my understanding of compassion?
- How do my cultural values and upbringing impact on the way I treat those who are suffering?
- Do I treat myself too harshly when I fail or am I able to be compassionate to myself?

In Chapters 2 and 3, we discovered how the notion of compassion was understood and explained by philosophers of different eras and different geographical areas in the world. We also explored how five major religions in the world explain and apply compassion. Many elements of compassion, such as that of the Golden Rule, appear to be accepted almost universally. Nursing codes of conduct as well as those of other healthcare professions expect practitioners to care with compassion, often explaining this in terms of kindness, dignity, human rights and personalised care. In contrast to the acceptance of certain universal principles of compassion, what is proposed in this book is that invariably these principles and meanings cannot be applied across all cultures without considering the specific circumstances and context.

However, the connection between culture and compassion in healthcare has hardly been studied. We may of course extrapolate knowledge from literature that looks at, for example, the impact of culture on health, health policy and practice (see Box 5.2), or from other disciplines such as psychology in terms of the nature and expression of emotions, or anthropology in terms of customs, rituals and worldviews, or sociology in terms of family structures and expressions of compassion and so on, but studies that focus specifically on the cultural aspects of compassion in health and illness and how these may be understood and dealt with by healthcare providers are extremely rare.

Papadopoulos and Pezzella (2015) conducted a study to investigate how compassion is embedded in the textbooks used in undergraduate mental health nursing degree courses. They found that none of the textbooks directly addressed the issue of compassion or culturally competent compassion. They concluded that this finding may reflect the lack of culturally based compassion knowledge and urged for more research and scholarly studies to be undertaken in order to develop learning tools to be used by students, teachers and practitioners.

Chambers and Ryder (2009) provide one of the few scholarly texts that attempts to connect culture, diversity and compassion. Through a number of case studies, they explore compassionate care through the prisms of culture, age, sexual orientation and so on. They express the view that in order to provide individualised care, healthcare workers must not only appreciate the diversity of their patients, but also understand that the patients' cultural norms and values can vary within seemingly homogeneous groups.

Recognising that cultural similarities and differences in the ways compassion is given and received between a nurse and a patient (including his or her family) can help the nurse and other healthcare givers seek to understand their patients' and families' cultural beliefs about compassion and how best to comfort them and the patient (see Box 5.3). Even if the nurse and the patient come from the same culture, they may not share the same understanding of what is appropriate compassion. However, it is less likely that care void of culturally competent compassion will be given if the nurse is aware of these facts and is able to verify with the family and/or the patient whether, for example, holding the hand of the patient or sharing the patient's sadness through an embrace are appropriate and acceptable.

Discussion about similarities and differences at the country level can be found in Chapter 8, which reports the results of an international study that explored and compared the meaning of compassion among nurses from fifteen countries.

(c) Cultural sensitivity and compassion

The third construct of culturally sensitive compassion is about developing culturally sensitive and compassionate therapeutic relationships. The suggested learning for this construct focuses

BOX 5.2 EXAMPLES OF CULTURAL BELIEFS AND COMPASSION

1. Female genital mutilation

It is often argued by the members of cultures that carry out female genital mutilation on young girls that this is a compassionate act. This is based on their belief that this would enable the girl to find a husband.

2. Disclosure of bad news

As a rule, Western societies believe that a person has the right to know the truth about their health status and doing so is considered a compassionate act. However, in many cultures, there exists the belief that it is unkind to tell someone that their illness is incurable and they may die soon. They believe that the family should be given such news first, and it is they will decide when, how and what they will disclose to the patient.

3. Health beliefs and the family

Although increasingly family structures and roles are changing in most societies, our clinical experiences tell us that families are important to most patients, albeit to different extents. Being compassionate to a member of one's family is demonstrated in different ways by different cultures and sometimes even by members of the same culture. Highly collectivist cultures believe that in a stressful situation, such as when one of their family members falls ill, treating each other with concern and compassion will be beneficial to the person who is ill. The family elders must be consulted and play a pivotal role at all stages of the person's illness.

For example, in the Gypsy Traveller community, the grandmother is the ultimate decision-maker when it comes to children's illness management.

Greek people express their compassion to someone who is ill by continuous visitations from family and friends. They believe that the constant presence by family members at the bedside demonstrates their love and support and provides encouragement to the sick person.

Ill members of individualist cultures are more likely to be in control of their own needs, rights and health goals. Close family members will most probably show their compassion by respecting the person's independence.

4. Eliminating pain

Although the very definition of culturally competent compassion speaks of the alleviation of suffering (which may be physical pain), not all cultures consider this as a desired goal. For example, suffering is a key aspect of Buddhism, and enduring it is a means of purification. The ways that the nurse may express her compassion in such situations may be in terms of being with the patient rather than focusing her/his efforts on alleviating the pain.

BOX 5.3 CULTURAL KNOWLEDGE AND COMPASSION REFLECTION ACTIVITY

Some relevant questions to reflect on are:

- Do I know how those whose cultural backgrounds are different from mine understand compassion?
- Do I know how similar their understanding is to mine?
- Do I know what are acceptable compassionate behaviours for those whose cultural backgrounds differ from my own?
- Am I open-minded and tolerant about the compassion values and behaviours of others?
- Can I challenge compassion beliefs and traditions that I disagree with?
- Is my reasoning regarding knowing and challenging motivated by the right desires?

BOX 5.4 CULTURAL SENSITIVITY AND COMPASSION REFLECTION ACTIVITY

Some relevant questions to reflect on are:

- How can I improve my communication so that I can express appropriate compassion in both verbal and non-verbal ways?
- Can I recognise the signs of emotional suffering in people whose cultural backgrounds are different to mine?
- How do I develop my practical wisdom to be able to know and do the right thing in a culturally and compassionately sensitive manner?
- How do I negotiate intercultural encounters to be able to deal with misunderstandings and conflict in a culturally and compassionately sensitive manner?

---

on the affective and relational aspects of culturally sensitive compassion. Important to this is a person's ability to communicate effectively and appropriately. The knowledge of what is and is not an acceptable way to give and receive compassion is crucial, as is the understanding of the non-verbal aspects of communication. We must learn not only what to communicate, but also how to communicate (see Box 5.4). For example, in many cultures, compassion is expressed through touch, such as handshakes and hugs. Srivastava (2007) explains that what is considered an appropriate amount of touch and personal space is determined by cultural norms and contexts. In cultures with greater personal distance such as India, non-touch greeting gestures such as bowing or holding one's hands in front of one's face in a prayer pose ('*namaste*') are used. Srivastava (2007) adds that touch is also used to convey respect and power, such as patting someone's back or putting an arm around another's shoulder. Gender and age rules also need to be taken into consideration when providing compassion through touch. It is considered highly inappropriate for a stranger, particularly a male stranger, to have physical contact with an Orthodox Jewish or a devout Muslim woman. Because of the individual differences between and within cultures, the most culturally sensitive approach to providing compassion through touch is by assessing and verifying – whilst using appropriate questioning – what is and is not culturally acceptable to a particular patient.

(d) Cultural competence and compassion

The final construct is that of culturally competent compassion, the definition of which was given previously. This stage is the synthesis of the previous three (awareness, knowledge and sensitivity) and their application in the real world (see Box 5.5). Health professionals are expected to be cognisant of human rights in order to champion these rights, but also to be courageous enough to challenge any violations of them. Linked to human rights and the aims of education for world citizenship, health professionals should have a sense of interconnectedness and belonging to the world community.

The above case study illustrates the consequences of culturally incompetent and compassionless care. The doctor obviously lacked a basic understanding of Ethiopian cultural beliefs and behaviours. He mistook Selassie's quiet demeanour and lack of directness in his limited communication as signs of depression. He dismissed the pain and fatigue as symptoms of depression rather than signs of a physical health problem and failed to engage

---

BOX 5.5 WHERE IS CULTURALLY COMPETENT COMPASSION?

Selassie is a forty-year-old man who has been living in the UK for nearly two and a half years. He comes from a rural part of Ethiopia. His speaks basic English and lives alone in a house that he shares with five other men from different cultural backgrounds. He feels lonely and is finding it difficult to adjust to living in the UK. About a year ago, he developed pain in the kidney area associated with fatigue. According to him, the doctor did not examine him, and as there was not an interpreter present, the doctor just gave him a prescription. Selassie took the medicine but the pain did not go away, so he returned several times to the doctor. Selassie did not know that he could ask for an interpreter to be present during the consultation and the doctor did not seemed interested in Selassie's explanation about his feelings and symptoms. About six months after the first consultation, Selassie develop acute pain, swelling, headaches and noticed blood in his urine. He decided to attend the accident and emergency department of the local hospital. He took his medication with him to show the nurses and doctors. After some tests, he was told that his medication was an anti-depressant and that one of his kidney was severely damaged and needed to be removed. Selassie is feeling better now, but he is sad that he had to lose one of his kidneys and believes that this happened because the doctor did not value him as a human being and that his actions were disrespectful and lacked compassion.

BOX 5.6 CULTURAL COMPETENCE AND COMPASSION REFLECTION ACTIVITY

Some relevant questions to reflect on are:

- Am I competently applying my cultural awareness, knowledge and sensitivity in my practice?
- Am I courageous enough to speak up and challenge injustice and human rights violations when I see them?
- Do I possess the practical wisdom to challenge constructively at the right time and through the right channels?
- Am I aware of the crises facing humankind and do I think about my contributions to relevant solutions?

---

an interpreter, which would have enabled him to delve deeper into Selassie's symptoms. The doctor also failed to question his original assumptions and diagnosis even after Selassie's return appointments. Coming from a high power distance culture where asking a doctor to explain the type and purpose of prescribed medication would have been viewed as a challenge to authority, Selassie did not do this even though his basic English would have been sufficient. The doctor's attitude as perceived by Selassie was dehumanising when it should have been compassionate. Notwithstanding the considerable waste of human and other resources used in dealing with Selassie, the result of culturally and compassionately incompetent care was much unnecessary suffering and the loss of a precious kidney.

In summary, the above case study highlighted the lack of the following elements that are crucial for culturally competent and compassionate care:

- Understanding my cultural values and beliefs and how these impact on my understanding of compassion
- Affording all human beings equal value and respect
- Having the motivation to learn about my patients' cultural health beliefs and behaviours
- Engaging with all patients through culturally sensitive and compassionate communication
- Having the humility to challenge my assumptions and question my actions
- Providing all patients equal access to care and treatments
- Utilising the available resources, such as interpreters, to benefit the patients who need them

The achievement of culturally competent compassion takes time, education, good role models, a clinical environment that promotes and nurtures compassion and lots of practice. This should not be viewed as something that we do when we have time. It should be integral to healthcare practice at all levels and in all contexts (see Box 5.6). As discussed in Chapter 1 of this book, ignoring this most important approach to providing care has resulted and will continue to result in much human suffering and avoidable costs.

Applications of the model

Theories and models can only become useful and impactful if the people they are aimed at become aware of their existence, learn how to use them and, crucially, if this learning is then put into practice. Exemplars of how models can help to promote learning can act as guidance to those who wish to use these theories and models. For this reason, I provide here two examples of how my colleagues and I have applied the Papadopoulos model described in this chapter.

(1) The pioneering massive online open course on cultural competence and compassion

I used this model to create the first massive online open course (MOOC) on culturally competent compassion, which was delivered at the end of 2014/beginning of 2015 and attended by 600 people from nearly 50 different countries. The MOOC was five weeks long and one week's worth of learning was assigned to each of the key constructs of the model. As the MOOC used democratic and active participatory methods of learning such as co-creation and collaborative learning communities, participants with different worldviews were able to engage in intercultural dialogue, exchanging and debating their different perspectives, connecting these to real-life situations and developing mutual respect. The participants of the MOOC (a mixture of health and social care workers and others) reported that they found learning together very interesting, thought-provoking and a challenging way of discovering similarities and differences between them. This MOOC provides an example of what can be done by higher education to promote the values and principles of culturally competent compassion and world citizenship.

(2) The Intercultural Education of Nurses in Europe programme

I mentioned earlier that the educational principles informing the Papadopoulos model for developing culturally competent compassion in healthcare professionals are those described in a book edited by Josef Huber in 2012 entitled *Intercultural competence for all: Preparing for living in a heterogeneous world*, which was published by the Council of Europe. I have combined those principles with others found in the wider literature on educating the world citizen to produce the following list, which was used during the Intercultural Education of Nurses in Europe (IENE) programme. Thus, intercultural education is about:

- Respecting the cultural background and identity of the learner by relating learning to their previous knowledge and experiences
- Providing equal access to learning by eliminating discrimination in the education system and by promoting an inclusive learning environment
- Promoting learning that encourages the understanding of personal values and the development of self-awareness, both of which form the basis for reflective communication and cooperation across cultures and social boundaries
- Promoting a critical approach regarding the potential of the power linked to the production and use of knowledge to either oppress or emancipate people
- Tolerating language imperfections by providing language support and/or by allowing extra time for people to express themselves
- Avoiding over-dependence on oral learning methods and using visual and other interactive and culturally appropriate learning approaches

- Emphasising realism – intercultural learning is a lifelong process
- Promoting courage – thinking outside the box and speaking out against injustice

My second example of culturally competent compassion in higher education comes from the IENE programme, which I have been coordinating since 2008. The third project of the IENE programme involved the participation of six European countries (the UK, Romania, Italy, The Netherlands, Germany and Turkey) in the development of three learning tools (IENE3 Tools, 2013–2015) covering the following topic areas of intercultural education:

Tool 1 – culturally competent compassion
Tool 2 – culturally competent courage
Tool 3 – intercultural communication

A total of 18 tools were produced and can all be found on the programme's multilingual website at www.ieneproject.eu.

Taken from the United Nations Human Rights Declaration, the overall guiding value of the IENE3 tool methodology was based on the powerful statement that I referred to in an earlier part of this chapter: "All human beings are born free and equal in dignity and rights. They are endowed with reason and conscience and should act towards one another in a spirit of brotherhood" (www.un.org/en/universal-declaration-human-rights). The other guiding values are those identified above in terms of intercultural education.

The content and activities for the tools were structured according to the Papadopoulos model of culturally competent compassion (Figure 5.2). The activities were innovative and thought-provoking, utilising presentations, games, songs, pictures, reading, videos, role-play, discussion, brainstorming and opportunities for reflective learning. Furthermore, a number of case studies were also included.

Following the piloting of the tools with student nurses, some very positive feedback was received, including the following:

- "Very nice and creative lesson. It really helps the teaching of cultural and compassionate issues."
- "It was wonderful to see how compassion care affected the students."
- "Learned a lot and I can really use it in my daily practice."
- "It was enlightening…every nurse can learn from this…"
- "An eye opener to use this way to ask questions, without prejudices."
- "Very instructive, I can use this in my daily practice."
- "Enjoyed being involved in collaborative learning."

Conclusions

Learning to become a culturally competent and compassionate human being is crucial in order to be able to cross cultural boundaries and develop effective interpersonal relations with people from diverse cultures. Intercultural education focusing on the virtues that underpin education for global citizenship should be driving university education. It is the right of every student to receive an education that will enable him/her to flourish and make a difference in the world, not only in terms of the economy and science, but also crucially in terms of finding ways to address conflict and help people live with others in a peaceful world where the humanity of every one of us is of equal worth, extending to a harmonious co–existence with non–humans and a respect for nature.

LEARNING ACTIVITY

Tahir's story

Tahir is transferred to your ward for observations. He is a young man who was brought into the accident and emergency department of the hospital by two friends at around 10 p.m. His friends explained that he was attacked in a city street by a gang of drunken youths who punched him to the ground and then proceeded to kick him. They were also attacked as they tried to protect their friend, but they could defend themselves, whilst Tahir could not do so once he was on the ground. He has been assessed and treated for head injuries because he was disorientated, with severe swelling around his eyes and bleeding from cuts on his face. He has been calling for his mother and also appears to be calling for Allah's help.

According to the information provided by his friends, Tahir is from Syria. He is sixteen years old and recently arrived in the UK through illegal people-smuggling operations. He speaks very little English and since his arrival he has been living rough, receiving some help from other refugees.

Caring for Tahir

Using the Papadopoulos model of culturally competent compassion and taking into consideration the information you have about Tahir and his condition, prepare a plan on how would you go about providing culturally competent and compassionate care to him. Ideally, you should plan for his immediate care whilst also making a contribution towards his long-term needs.

References

Baughan, J. and Smith, A. (2013). *Compassion, caring and communication. Skills for nursing practice.* 2nd Ed. Abingdon, UK: Routledge.

Chambers, C. and Ryder, E. (2009). *Compassion and caring in nursing.* Abingdon, UK: Radcliffe Publishing Ltd.

Chochinov, J. (2007). Dignity and the essence of medicine: The A, B, C and D of dignity conserving care. *BMJ*, 63, pp. 184–187.

Cummings, J. and Bennett, V. (2012). Developing the culture of compassionate care. Creating a new vision for nurses, midwives and care-givers. NHS Commissioning Board. Retrieved January 2018 from: www.england.nhs.uk/wp-content/uploads/2012/12/compassion-in-practice.pdf.

Department of Health (2009). *The NHS constitution: The NHS belongs to us all.* London, UK: Department of Health.

Delors, J., ed. (1996). *Learning: The treasure within. Report to UNESCO of the Task Force on Education for the Twenty-first Century.* Paris, France, UNESCO Publishing.

Francis, R. and The Mid Staffordshire NHS Foundation Trust Inquiry (2010). *The independent inquiry into care provided by Mid Staffordshire NHS Foundation Trust January 2005–March 2009.* London, UK: The Stationary Office.

Frank, A.W. (2004). *The renewal of generosity: Illness, medicine and how to live.* Chicago, IL: The University of Chicago Press.

Goetz, J.L., Keltner, F. and Simon-Thomas, E. (2010). Compassion: An evolutionary analysis and empirical review. Psychological Bulletin, 136(3), pp. 351–374.

Hall, S. and Jefferson, T., eds (1996). *Resistance through rituals: Youth sub-culture in post-war Britain.* London, UK: Hutchinson.

Hewison, A. and Sawbridge, Y. (2016). *Compassion in nursing. Theory, evidence and practice.* London, UK: Palgrave

Huber, J., ed. (2012). *Intercultural competence for all. Preparation for living in a heterogeneous world.* Strasbourg, France: Council of Europe Publishing.

Firth-Cozens, J. and Cornwell, J. (2009). *The point of care. Enabling compassionate care in acute hospital settings.* London, UK: Kings Fund.

Lowenstein, J. (2008). *The midnight meal and other essays about doctors, patients, and medicine.* New Haven, CT: Yale University Press.

Neff, K. (2011). Self-compassion, self-esteem, and well-being. *Social and Personality Psychology Compass,* 5(1), pp. 1–12.

Papadopoulos, I., Tilki, M. and Taylor, G. (1998). *Transcultural care. A guide for health care professionals.* Dinton, UK: Quay Publications.

Papadopoulos, I., ed. (2006). *Transcultural health and social care: Development of culturally competent practitioners.* Edinburgh, UK: Churchill Livingstone Elsevier.

Papadopoulos, I. (2011). *Courage, compassion and cultural competence.* Paper presented at the 13th Anna Reynvaan Lecture. De Stadsschouwburg – Amsterdam City Theatre, The Netherlands.

Papadopoulos, I. (2014). The Papadopoulos model for developing culturally competent compassion in healthcare professionals. Retrieved November 2016 from: www.youtube.com/watch?v=zjKzO94TevA.

Papadopoulos, I. and Pezzella, A. (2015). A snapshot review of culturally competent compassion as addressed in selected mental health textbooks for undergraduate nursing students. Journal of Compassionate Health *Care*, 2, 3.

Papadopoulos, I., Taylor, G., Ali, S., Aagard, M., Akman, O., Alpers, L.M., …, Zorba, A. (2017). Exploring nurses' meaning and experiences of compassion: An international online survey involving 15 countries. *Journal of Transcultural Nursing,* 28(3), pp. 286–295.

Papadopoulos, I., Zorba, A., Koulouglioti, C., Ali, S., Aagard, M., Akman, O., …, Vasiliou, M. (2016). International study on nurses' views and experiences of compassion. *International Nursing Review,* 63(3), pp. 395–405.

Sellman, D. (2011). *What makes a good nurse.* London, UK: Jessica Kingsley Publishers.

Shea, S., Wynyard, R. and Lionis, C., eds (2014). *Providing compassionate healthcare. Challenges in policy and practice.* Abingdon, UK: Routledge.

Srivastava, R.H., ed. (2007). *The healthcare professional's guide to clinical cultural competence.* Toronto, Canada: Mosby Elsevier Canada.

Strauss, C., Taylor, B.L., Gu, J., Kuyken, W., Baer, R., Jones, F. and Cavanagh, K. (2016). What is compassion and how can we measure it? A review of definitions and measures. *Clinical Psychology Review,* 47, pp. 15–27.

Tilki, M. (2006). Human rights and health inequalities: UK and EU policies and initiatives relating to the promotion of culturally competent care. In: I. Papadopoulos, ed. *Transcultural health and social care: Development of culturally competent practitioners.* Edinburgh, UK: Churchill Livingstone Elsevier, pp. 25–43.

UNESCO (2014). Learning to live together. Paris, France and Bangkok, Thailand, UNESCO Publishing.

UN General Assembly (1948). Universal Declaration of Human Rights, 10 December 1948, 217 A (III), Paris.

van der Cingel, M. (2011). Compassion in care: A qualitative study of older people with a chronic disease and nurses. Nursing Ethics, 18(5), pp. 672–685.

6

LEARNING AND PRACTISING CULTURALLY COMPETENT COMPASSION

LEARNING OBJECTIVES

Upon completion of this chapter, readers should be able to:

- Understand the need for culturally competent compassion.
- Discuss the barriers to theoretical learning of culturally competent compassion.
- Outline solutions and suggestions on how culturally competent compassion can be learnt.
- Appreciate the importance of practice-based learning and the need for good role models.
- Understand the importance of practical wisdom and how to develop it.

Introduction

The question as to whether compassion can be taught/learned and how has been a subject of some debate in recent years (Adamson and Dewar, 2011; Curtis, 2013). Instinctively, many people, including healthcare professionals, respond that one is either compassionate or is not, and therefore compassion cannot be taught (Barker, 2013). At the same time, this view is qualified by stating that one adopts compassionate values and behaviours from early childhood, with the mother's love being the first stimulus that plants the seed of compassion in a person. Recent developments in neuropsychology and neurobiology provide evidence that our brains possess a complex system of neurons providing the potential for compassion and compassionate behaviours. Further, it is asserted that compassionate behaviours and emotions can be learned. Ashar, et al. (2016) provide an excellent account of the factors that come into play in order to activate our innate potential for compassion and the benefits of it for ourselves and others. As discussed in Chapters 2 and 3 of this book, many philosophers and religions profess that compassion is an essential human value or virtue that should be promoted through learning by example, as well as through reading and self-reflection.

There is now sufficient evidence that teaching, learning and assessing compassion within healthcare should be part of the process of lifelong learning, together with the need to encourage suitable role models (Shea, et al., 2014; Papadopoulos, et al., 2016). In the UK, various government-commissioned reports (Francis, 2010; Berwick, 2013; Keogh, 2013) include recommendations for nursing education and the education of other health professionals that make the inclusion of compassion in their curricula an inescapable challenge, whilst the Nursing and Midwifery Council's new Code of Practice (NMC, 2015) requires that nurses treat people with kindness, respect and compassion. The NHS Constitution (2015, p.5) also strongly emphasises compassion by stating that:

> We ensure that compassion is central to the care we provide and respond with humanity and kindness to each person's pain, distress, anxiety or need. We search for the things we can do, however small, to give comfort and relieve suffering. We find time for patients, their families and carers, as well as those we work alongside. We do not wait to be asked, because we care.

This is a profound statement that establishes beyond any doubt the right of each patient and each health worker to be treated with compassion.

The position taken in this book is that compassion is a virtue to be cultivated (Aristotle, 384–322 BCE; Bradshaw, 2009). Furthermore, as has been highlighted in Chapter 1 and repeated in other chapters, this book's focus is on culturally competent compassion in recognition of the fact that the enactment of compassion varies from culture to culture. Examples of specific cultural differences that impact on compassion and need to be taken into consideration when learning to provide culturally competent and compassionate care are the notions of time, being there, going the extra mile, defending and advocating and personalisation of care (Papadopoulos, et al., 2017). Societies across the globe are and will continue to be multicultural, a fact that is increasingly recognised by governments and national and international regulatory bodies that are expecting health service providers to be culturally competent. For example, in 2014, the International Council of Nurses endorsed the guidelines for implementing culturally competent nursing care (Douglas, et al., 2014).

Classroom-based teaching

Despite the clear evidence of the need to educate nurses to be culturally competent and compassionate, an international survey involving 1323 respondents from fifteen countries reported that although more than half (59.6%) of them felt that compassion could be taught to nurses, 44.3% of them stated that not enough teaching about compassion is provided (Papadopoulos, et al., 2016).

Barriers to theoretical learning

Why do so many nurses in different countries report that not enough teaching about compassion is provided? Let us briefly address some of the reasons and barriers as well as examples of good practice (Box 6.1).

BOX 6.1 CULTURALLY COMPETENT AND COMPASSIONATE CARE

Barriers to theoretical learning	_Solutions and examples of good practice_
(a) Teachers' and students' values and beliefs	(a) The point of care (King's Fund)
(b) Lack of teachers' competence in the topic	(b) Support teachers to develop self-compassion (Neff, 2011)
(c) Lack of resources for teachers and students	(c) The IENE3 programme: tools for compassion (Brown, 2014; Adamson and Smith, 2014; Chambers and Ryder, 2009)
(d) Lack of suitable models and frameworks to systematically plan and deliver it	(d) The Papadopoulos model of culturally competent compassion (2014)

Teachers' and students' values and beliefs

We have already explored the belief that compassion cannot be taught because we either naturally have it or do not have it. Another contestable belief is that if one is caring for a patient then he/she is also being compassionate. Therefore, if students study 'caring', they are learning about compassion. In an ideal world, this should be the case. However, caring is often reduced to a set of clinical procedures and tasks that can be taught and performed without the relational and emotional component that is compassion. Firth-Cozens and Cornwell (2009) in their King's Fund report entitled _The point of care: Enabling compassionate care in acute hospital settings_ emphasised that although aspects of compassion feature in the curricula of most healthcare professions, in medicine and increasingly in nursing, the curricula adhere to the biomedical model and evidenced-based practice, which tend to objectify patients, thus failing to see the person in the patient, a dehumanising process that has no place in nursing.

It is understandable that undergraduate students focus their efforts on acquiring the knowledge and skills that will enable them to be successful in their assessments/exams, most of which centre on facts and procedures about physical and psychological illnesses, nursing diagnoses and nursing interventions. The current nature of assessments may inadvertently undermine the value of compassion, even though this is enshrined in government reports and nursing codes of practice.

Lack of teachers' competence in the topic

Many teachers will agree with Frank's (2004) assertions that compassion is more than just acts of basic care, as it involves 'real dialogue' with the patients and their significant others. Real dialogue goes beyond communication and requires courage; it is an interaction with real interest between humans that recognises and celebrates their differences whilst appreciating their common core humanity.

According to the Papadopoulos (2014) model for developing culturally competent compassion, the starting point of this lifelong process is an awareness of our cultural identity and the need for self-compassion. Self-compassion, according to Neff (2011), involves treating ourselves with kindness, caring, nurturance and concern, rather than being harshly judgemental or indifferent to our suffering and vulnerabilities.

When we consider the issues we have discussed so far and the growing literature on the many facets of compassion as well as those of cultural competence, we may conclude that it is unlikely that many nursing teachers (or indeed teachers of other health professions) have been adequately prepared to plan and deliver culturally competent compassion beyond a superficial level. It is therefore urgent that teacher preparation is addressed rather than merely assumed. Governments and national and international nursing bodies have provided ambitious plans and promises – now we must find ways to deliver them.

Lack of resources for teachers and students

A range of teaching and learning methods are gradually emerging through a small number of expert facilitators who have run and evaluated courses on compassion. For example, Brown (2014) recommends experiential learning, group learning, imaginative writing, compassionate listening, visualisation and meditation.

Adamson and Smith (2014) recommend listening to patients' stories and using case studies, creative art and reflection. Chambers and Ryder (2009) also use case studies and reflection. Others suggest that learning via a multidisciplinary approach and exposure to the humanities, social sciences and art can represent positive ways forward by helping students to imagine the lives of others (Chochinov, 2007; Haslam, 2015).

I have used online learning in the form of a massive open online course on culturally competent compassion, making use of a range of activities involving video, written materials, discussion boards, quizzes and so on, enabling individual learning and learning communities (Papadopoulos, 2014). In addition, the IENE3 project that I coordinated produced comprehensive compassion tools available in different languages and open access at www. ieneproject.eu.

However, a snapshot review of the key mental health textbooks used in undergraduate curricula in the UK found that culturally competent compassion is not directly addressed in them (Papadopoulos and Pezzella, 2015). Although teachers and students have access to online resources and published articles, textbooks remain the key reference points for many students; therefore, it could be argued that this omission is negatively impacting on students' preparation to provide culturally competent and compassionate care.

The reviewed textbooks argued that, despite the universal nature of the emotions and behaviours associated with compassion, they are not all equally valued by cultures and religions. It is therefore important that students are encouraged to learn about and discuss the similarities and differences that exist between cultures in the way compassion is understood and expressed. This will help them establish sensitive and culturally appropriate compassionate relationships with the patients in their care. Since the notion of culturally competent compassion is fairly new (Papadopoulos, 2011), it is not surprising that teachers need more resources in order to be more effective at teaching it.

Lack of suitable models and frameworks to systematically plan and deliver culturally competent compassion

For change to happen, we need a strong argument, a wise leader and a roadmap that is easily understood and owned by its followers. The roadmap must provide just enough information so that it does not stifle the creativity of its followers and it must be flexible enough to adapt to different terrain. The roadmap should not be a standalone plan, but must connect and be part of other roadmaps whilst at the same time having a clear destination. To achieve the needed change in nursing education and to establish culturally competent compassion at its heart, a roadmap that meets the above criteria is required. I have developed such a roadmap – the Papadopoulos model for developing culturally competent and compassionate health professionals – which was presented in Chapter 5.

Practice-based learning

Learning through practice is most important not only for the undergraduate student, but for all who practice nursing. As discussed in Chapter 2, the Greek philosopher Aristotle (384–322 BCE) identified compassion as one of the most important human virtues and, according to him, the best way to attain it is through practice.

Fernando and Consedine (2014) explored the challenges to compassionate practice and found the following barriers:

- Burnout or overload, mainly due to time pressures
- External distractions, including bureaucratic requirements
- 'Difficult' patients and families
- Complex clinical situations, including uncertainty and failure of treatment

The same authors reported that intrinsic motivation (having a purpose, autonomy, related-ness and competence) is the key facilitator of compassionate practice. When this is nurtured, compassionate patient-centred care can flourish. Self-compassion is the key ingredient for the resilience a nurse needs in order to sustain her/his compassionate practice. Fernando and Consedine (2014) concluded that the nurturance of compassionate practice requires com-passionate leaders who embody and enact the virtues of altruism, integrity and humility and who are wise enough to appreciate the value of role modelling, empowering, supporting and enabling staff and patients to flourish.

The need for role modelling

It is clear from what we have discussed so far that learning from theoretical perspectives alone is unlikely to represent a sufficient means of instilling the virtue of compassion and encouraging the sustainability of culturally competent compassion throughout one's profes-sional practice. Ultimately, the aim is to be able to provide healthcare that takes into account peoples' cultural beliefs, behaviours and needs, whilst at the same time healthcare providers must develop the skills to reflect on how their own cultural backgrounds may influence their professional attitudes and practices.

Reinforcing and building upon what is learned in the classroom through practice and reflection is essential – as with any skill in life, the more we practice, the better we become.

For student nurses, the quality of their practice placements represents a good starting point for the development of culturally competent and compassionate caring skills. NHS Employers (2017) quote the editor of *Nursing Times*, Jenni Middleton, who stated during the 2013 annual Student Nursing Times award that:

Students tell us over and over again that their placement is one of the most important aspects of their training. A positive placement experience will not only teach good practice but will also coach students in how to develop relationships with their peers and patients. Student nurses often approach their placements with a certain amount of trepidation, but our finalists [the annual Student Nursing Times Awards] have created cultures that are supportive, caring and empathetic – the best environments in which to nurture the next generation of nursing talent. We applaud their positivity, enthusiasm and wisdom.

Practical wisdom

Cruess, Cruess and Steinert (2008) suggest that the characteristics of good role models are as follows:

- Clinical competence: this is integral to practice and needs to be role modelled. It includes clinical reasoning and decision-making, knowledge and skills and communication.
- Teaching skills: these are tools that are essential to role modelling in order to acquire clinical competence, including effective communication and opportunities for reflection.
- Personal qualities: there are a number of attributes that contribute to role modelling. These include a commitment to best practice as well as being motivated and enthusiastic about teaching and practising, as well as having interpersonal relationship skills.

I would like to add one more category. Some of the elements of my category are implied in the three categories above, but this is not enough. In my view, good role models, especially those who promote culturally competent compassion, possess practical wisdom.

According to Aristotle (Crisp, 2014), practical wisdom (phronesis) is the virtue of practical reasoning. Practical reasoning allows us to investigate what we can change and helps us to make good choices. In order to make good choices, not only must our reasoning be correct, but we must also have the right desires. The person with practical wisdom not only uses it for their professional work, but crucially, she or he uses it to reason about how to live a good life. Practical wisdom differs from other sorts of knowledge because of both its complexity and its practical nature. Aristotle claimed that practical wisdom involves:

- A general conception of what is good or bad related to the conditions for human flourishing
- The ability to perceive, in light of that general conception, what is required in terms of feeling, choice and action in a particular situation
- The ability to deliberate well
- The ability to act on that deliberation

Phronesis, then, involves general knowledge, particular knowledge (a relevant example here would be the particular cultural enactments of compassion), an ability to reason regarding a choice and an ability to act on that choice.

Most nurse practitioners and leaders would agree that the components of compassion listed in Figure 8.1 are all linked to doing the right thing. However, not all of them would know how to balance the clashing demands between one right thing and another. This requires practical wisdom.

Many decisions in healthcare involve high levels of moral reasoning. This is the heart of practical wisdom, and a good role model understands that moral knowledge is only acquired through experience. A good role model applies practical wisdom by combining the will to do the right thing with the skill to figure out what the right thing is. Students and novice practitioners can learn from role models with practical wisdom on how, for example, to balance the desire to spend enough time with a patient in order to be thorough, compassionate and understanding with the need to see other patients who also require her/his help. An experienced role model will demonstrate the golden mean, a characteristic of practical wisdom that enables us to learn to succeed at our practices and to flourish as human beings. For example, a nurse can give too much, too little or no culturally competent compassion. None of these states are desirable. Too much culturally competent compassion – such as feeling as much suffering as the patient – will render the nurse unable to help the patient. Too little or no culturally competent compassion dehumanises the patient, resulting in more suffering. An experienced role model using her/his practical wisdom and the reasoning abilities inherent in it will choose the right amount of compassion, something that Aristotle called the golden mean.

Leaders as role models

The successful achievement of ongoing learning through practice is partially dependent on the skills of leaders within and across the organisation who possess practical wisdom, can demonstrate a commitment to ethical and professional values and can influence the establishment of nurturing environments (see Chapter 7).

In a study by Dauvrin and Lorant (2015), an investigation into the influence of leaders on the cultural competence of healthcare professionals demonstrated that the health professionals' own competence was associated with the cultural competence of their leaders.

McSherry, et al. (2012) suggest that the challenge facing the nursing profession is ensuring that the core principles of dignity, respect, compassion and person-centred care become central to all aspects of nursing practice. Excellence in nursing care will happen if nurse managers, leaders and educators are able to respond to the complexity of reform and change by enabling, empowering and encouraging staff and by inspiring them through their own deeds and behaviours.

Despite the many benefits of role modelling in practice, Baldwin, et al. (2014) draw attention to the fact that this remains an undervalued learning experience that should be brought to the forefront of discussions, particularly in relation to undergraduate nursing education. It would seem logical that if a student is able to systematically observe a leader or colleague who is performing with compassion, cultural competence and clinical excellence and is then encouraged to apply the skills she/he observed as well as reflect on them, the benefits will be enormous.

Exposure to practical wisdom through role modelling can enhance the learning experience for students and better equip them for the unpredictability of patient care. Effective role modelling can nurture and assist in the development and sustainability of care that is professional, humanistic, compassionate and culturally competent. Furthermore, role modelling can help to encourage self-care and resilience and the development of self-compassion.

SUMMARY

- The position taken in this book is that compassion is a virtue to be cultivated (Aristotle, 384–322 BCE; Bradshaw, 2009).
- There is now sufficient evidence that teaching, learning and assessing compassion within healthcare should be part of the process of lifelong learning, together with the need to encourage suitable role models (Shea, et al., 2014; Papadopoulos, et al., 2016).
- Current barriers perceived by teachers prevent nursing students and qualified nurses from learning the praxis of culturally competent compassion.
- A number of research and/or practice-based solutions that address the barriers are provided in this chapter.
- Nursing and other health professions need to have culturally competent and compassionate role models in order to promote and nurture culturally competent and compassionate clinical practice.

LEARNING ACTIVITY

Scenario: The complexities of care and how practical wisdom can help

Megan Jones is a thirty-nine-year-old nurse in charge of a surgical ward. Today, she is working with Anne Smith, a second-year student nurse. They are looking after Mrs Ahmed, a seventy-year-old lady originally from Pakistan, who is alert and speaks English well. She was admitted to the ward three days ago for investigations regarding several episodes of rectal bleeding, pain and weight loss and is in a side room on her own. She has had several blood tests and a biopsy and the results have just arrived. She has bowel cancer. Mrs Ahmed asks Megan to give her the results of her tests. Megan knows that Mrs Ahmed has the right to know her diagnosis, but at the same time she is aware that Mrs Ahmed's family have asked that they are told the results before her. Megan understands that the family is trying to protect Mrs Ahmed from hearing the bad news from a nurse or a doctor. They believe that they can present the news in a more hopeful and compassionate way than the ward staff. Megan acknowledges that she is in a difficult position. She wants to do the right thing. As Mrs Ahmed is adamant that she wants to know her results, and since Megan knows that the patient is an intelligent woman who speaks good English, she decides to do the right thing for the patient. She closes the room door, sits on Mrs Ahmed's bed and, whilst holding her hand and in the presence of Anne, she proceeds to tell her the bad news in a compassionate manner. Megan answers Mrs Ahmed's questions truthfully and compassionately. Mrs Ahmed begins to cry and Megan offers her some tissues. Whilst embracing Mrs Ahmed, she feels emotional, sharing her grief.

She then asks Mrs Ahmed if she wants her to call her son and whether she wants to be alone to pray. Mrs Ahmed explains that there is no need to telephone her son as he is due to visit later on. Megan leaves Mrs Ahmed to pray whilst informing her that she can speak to the doctor about her treatment options any time she is ready.

Questions:

- What role modelling approaches did Megan adopt?
- Describe the practical wisdom abilities that Megan used.
- Was this experience useful to Anne and why?

Later that day, Mrs Ahmed's son visits to find his mother upset. She tells him that the nurse in charge has informed her that she has cancer. He storms out of the room into Megan's office, shouting at her because she did not follow his instructions.

Questions:

- How should Megan approach her meeting with Mr Ahmed?
- Consider the cultural and ethical issues in this scenario.
- How should Megan deal with Mr Ahmed in order to provide a positive role model to Anne?

References

Adamson, E. and Dewar, B. (2011). Compassion in the nursing curriculum: Making it more explicit. *Journal of Holistic Healthcare*, 8, pp. 42–45.

Adamson, L. and Smith, S. (2014). Can compassion be taught? Experiences from the leadership in Compassionate Care Programme, Edinburgh Napier University and NHS Lothian. In: S. Shea, R. Wynyard and C. Lionis, eds. *Providing compassionate healthcare. Challenges in policy and practice*. Abingdon, UK: Routledge, pp. 235–251.

Ashar, Y.K., Andrews-Hanna, J.R., Dimidjian, S. and Wager, T.D. (2016). Toward a neuroscience of compassion: A brain systems-based model and research agenda. In: J.D. Greene, I. Morrison and M.E.P. Seligman, eds. *Positive neuroscience*. New York, NY: Oxford University Press, pp. 125–142.

Baldwin, A., Jane Mills, J., Birks, M. and Budde, L. (2014). Role modeling in undergraduate nursing education: An integrative literature review. *Nurse Education Today*, 34, pp. e18–e26.

Barker, K. (2013). Can care and compassion be taught? *British Journal of Midwifery*, 21, 82.

Berwick, D. (2013). *Berwick review into patient safety*. London, UK: Department of Health. Retrieved from: www.gov.uk/government/publications/berwick-review-into-patient-safety.

Bradshaw, A. (2009). Measuring nursing care and compassion: The McDonaldised nurse? *Journal of Medical Ethics*, 35, pp. 465–468.

Brown, C. (2014). Experiential learning and compassionate care. Encouraging changes in values, beliefs and behaviours. In: S. Shea, R. Wynyard and C. Lionis, eds. *Providing compassionate healthcare. Challenges in policy and practice*. Abingdon, UK: Routledge, pp. 54–67.

Chambers, C. and Ryder, E. (2009). *Compassion and caring in nursing*. Abingdon, UK: Radcliffe Publishing Ltd.

Chochinov, J. (2007). Dignity and the essence of medicine: The A, B, C and D of dignity conserving care. *British Medical Journal*, 63, pp. 184–187.

Crisp, R. (2014). *Artistotle: Nichomachean ethics*. Cambridge, UK: Cambridge University Press.

Cruess, S.R., Cruess, R. and Steinert, Y. (2008). Role modelling – Making the most of a powerful teaching strategy. *British Medical Journal*, 336, pp. 718–721.

Curtis, K. (2013). 21st century challenges faced by nursing faculty in educating for compassionate practice: Embodied interpretation of phenomenological data. *Nurse Education Today*, 33, pp. 746–750.

Dauvrin, M. and Lorant, V. (2015). Leadership and cultural competence of healthcare professionals: A social network analysis. *Nursing Research*, 64, pp. 200–210.

Department of Health (2015). The NHS Constitution for England. Retrieved from www.gov.uk/government/publications/the-nhs-constitution-for-england/the-nhs-constitution-for-england.

Douglas, M.K., Rosenkoetter, M., Pacquiao, D.F., Callister, L.C., Hattar-Pollara, M., Lauderdale, J., …, Purnell, L. (2014). Guidelines for implementing culturally competent nursing care. *Journal of Transcultural Nursing*, 25, pp. 109–121.

Fernando, A.T. and Considine, N.S. (2014). Beyond compassion fatigue: Development and preliminary validation of the Barriers to Physician Compassion Questionnaire. *Postgraduate Medical Journal*, 90, pp. 388–395.

Firth-Cozens, J. and Cornwell, J. (2009). *The point of care. Enabling compassionate care in acute hospital settings.* London, UK: Kings Fund.

Francis, R. (2010). *The Mid Staffordshire NHS Foundation Trust Inquiry. The independent inquiry into care provided by Mid Staffordshire NHS Foundation Trust January 2005–March 2009.* London, UK: The Stationery Office.

Frank, A.W. (2004). *The renewal of generosity: Illness, medicine and how to live.* Chicago, IL: The University of Chicago Press.

Haslam, D. (2015). More than kindness. *Journal of Compassionate Health Care*, 2, pp. 6–8.

Keogh, B. (2013). *Review into the quality of care and treatment provided by 14 hospital trusts in England: overview report.* London, UK: NHS England. Retrieved from: www.nhs.uk/nhsengland/bruce-keogh-review/documents/outcomes/keogh-review-final-report.pdf.

McSherry, R., Pearce, P., Grimwood, K. and McSherry, W. (2012). The pivotal role of nurse managers, leaders and educators in enabling excellence in nursing care. *Journal of Nursing Management*, 20, pp. 7–19.

Neff, K. (2011). Self-compassion, self-esteem, and well-being. *Social and Personality Psychology Compass*, 5, pp. 1–12.

NHS (2015). *The NHS constitution. The NHS belongs to us all.* London, UK: Crown Copyright.

NHS Employers (2017). Excellence in student nursing placements. Retrieved January 2018 from: www.nhsemployers.org/your-workforce/plan/nursing-workforce/nursing-education-and-training/excellence-in-student-nursing-placements.

Nursing and Midwifery Council (2015). *The Code: Professional standards of practice and behaviour for nurses and midwives.* London, UK: Nursing Midwifery Council. Retrieved from: www.nmc.org.uk/standards/code.

Papadopoulos, I., ed. (2006). *Transcultural health and social care: Development of culturally competent practitioners.* Edinburgh, UK: Churchill Livingstone Elsevier.

Papadopoulos, I. (2011). *Courage, compassion and cultural competence.* Paper presented at the 13th Anna Reynvaan Lecture. De Stadsschouwburg – Amsterdam City Theatre, The Netherlands.

Papadopoulos, I. (2014). The Papadopoulos model for developing culturally competent compassion in healthcare professionals. Retrieved November 2016 from: www.youtube.com/watch?v=zjKzO94TevA.

Papadopoulos, I. (in press). Intercultural compassion in higher education. In: P. Gibbs, ed. *The pedagogy of compassion at the heart of higher education.* New York, NY: Springer, pp. 73–84.

Papadopoulos, I. and Pezzella, A. (2015). A snapshot review of culturally competent compassion as addressed in selected mental health textbooks for undergraduate nursing students. *Journal of Compassionate Health Care*, 2, pp. 3–9.

Papadopoulos, I., Taylor, G., Ali, S., Aagard, M., Akman, O., Lise-Merete, A., …, Zorba, A. (2017). Exploring nurses' meaning and experiences of compassion: an international online survey involving 15 countries. *Journal of Transcultural Nursing*, 28, pp. 286–295.

Papadopoulos, I., Tilki, M. and Taylor, G. (1998). *Transcultural care. A guide for health care professionals.* Dinton, UK: Quay Publications.

Papadopoulos, I., Zorba, A., Koulouglioti, C., Ali, S., Aagard, M., Akman, O., …, Vasiliou, M. (2016). International study on nurses' views and experiences of compassion. *International Nursing Review*, 63, pp. 395–405.

Shea, S., Wynyard, R. and Lionis, C., eds (2014). *Providing compassionate healthcare. Challenges in policy and practice.* Abingdon, UK: Routledge.

7

CULTURALLY COMPETENT AND COMPASSIONATE LEADERSHIP

LEARNING OBJECTIVES

Upon completion of this chapter, readers should be able to:

- Appreciate the desirability of culturally competent and virtuous leadership.
- List the components of culturally competent and virtuous leadership.
- Distinguish between leaders and leadership.
- Have awareness of the IENE4 leadership resources.

Introduction

> We know when we see a leader. They inspire us and when we're inspired we become determined. And when we are determined we go further. That's what leadership is about…And it's your example that counts, not your rank. And if you care about patients to the point of being selfless, people will always respect that.
>
> *(Halligan, 2014)*

The quotation introducing this chapter consists of wise words by the late Aidan Halligan highlighting what connects practical wisdom and a genuine interest in our fellow humans to leadership. This chapter will look at leadership in nursing and in healthcare professions in general from a culturally competent, virtue-based perspective. We will consider why 'culturally competent virtuous leadership' is desirable and appropriate to healthcare professions.

What is leadership?

The King's Fund (2011) report entitled *The future of leadership and management in the NHS. No more heroes report* defined leadership as the art of motivating a group of people to achieve a common goal. A report published by the National Centre for Ethics in Health Care (Cook, et al., 2015) states that a key responsibility in leadership is ensuring that the organisation encourages employees to 'do the right thing'. As such, leaders should foster an environment and an organisational culture that supports doing the right thing and doing it well, for reasons that are supported by ethical values.

The Faculty of Medical Leadership and Management, The King's Fund and the Center for Creative Leadership (West, et al., 2015) collectively initiated a review of the evidence for leadership, the findings of which are summarised as follows:

- Leadership is required to ensure the delivery of high-quality and compassionate patient care.
- Leadership is required to develop inspiring visions operationalised at every level.
- Leadership is required to embody support for staff, honesty, kindness, altruism, fairness, accountability and optimism.
- Leadership is required to establish cultures that are not preoccupied with target setting, rules, regulations and status hierarchies.
- Leadership is most effective when all staff accept responsibility for their leadership roles, especially doctors, nurses and other clinicians.
- Leadership requires leaders to work together, spanning organisational boundaries both within and between organisations, prioritising overall patient care and working collectively to build a cooperative, integrative collective leadership culture.
- Experience in leadership is the most valuable factor in enabling leaders to develop their skills, especially when they have appropriate guidance and support. Focusing on how to enhance leaders' learning from experience should be a priority.
- National-level leadership is required to ensure that the overarching national organisations (Monitor, Care Quality Commission, NHS England and NHS Trust Development Authority) exemplify models of collective leadership, have positive cultures and have a core orientation of compassion towards the entire health service.

Why culturally competent virtuous leadership?

The findings of this extensive review indicate that there are different levels of leadership: national, organisational, unit/team and individual. The findings clearly emphasise that leadership is an ethical activity that should be founded on virtues such as compassion, honesty, kindness, fairness, altruism and cooperation. The importance of learning through experience and appropriate support and guidance strongly reminds us that nursing and other healthcare professions are practical professions and effective leaders need to have and use practical wisdom (see also Chapter 6).

In considering the nature of ethical leadership in nursing, Gallagher and Tschudin (2010) argue that all members of the nursing workforce are ethical leaders in so far as they demonstrate a commitment to ethical practice in their everyday work and act as ethical role models for others. Nurse managers are responsible for influencing their teams and for acting as arbiters between organisational and professional values.

Sellman (2011, pp. 17–18) suggests that "nursing is an inherently moral practice and that this places moral obligations on individual nurses to cultivate the sorts of dispositions necessary to ensure that nursing actions enable rather than diminish human flourishing." As a practice, nursing must cultivate the virtue of practical wisdom (phronesis), as this is the virtue by which all other virtues (those of the intellect and of the character) are given appropriate expression. According to Aristotle (384–322 BCE), practical wisdom is the ability to do the right thing at the right time and for the right reasons.

Papadopoulos (2006) points out that two of the underpinning pillars of transcultural nursing[1] and cultural competence are ethics and human rights. This is particularly important as transcultural nursing highlights two major challenges of the twenty-first century: (a) the multicultural nature of modern societies; and (b) the growing health inequalities.

Gallagher (2006) states that cultural misunderstandings and language differences may generate ethical dilemmas when healthcare providers lack the awareness of the value systems of patients that differ from their own. Goode and Like (2012) argue that strong and informed leadership is required in order to achieving patient services that are culturally and linguistically competent. They recommend that leadership should ensure that:

- Cultural and linguistic competence is cultivated at all levels of healthcare organisations and systems.
- The role of leaders must be revisited and adapted to address ongoing and emerging challenges: organisational change processes, differences across and within cultures and resulting dynamics, resistance and power differentials.

In the UK, the NHS Leadership Academy, which was set up in 2012 as one of the government's responses to addressing leadership issues identified in the Francis report (2010), aims to lead on making 'inclusion' a reality within the NHS through investment in excellent, knowledgeable and capable leadership. The Leadership Academy recognises that diversity and inclusion lead to improved health and more positive staff and patient experiences of the NHS (www.leadershipacademy.nhs.uk/resources/inclusion-equality-and-diversity).

The Leadership Academy's focus on inclusion is clearly linked to the following NHS England's statement:

> Promoting equality and equity are at the heart of our values – ensuring that we exercise fairness in all that we do and that no community or group is left behind in the improvements that will be made to health outcomes across the country.
>
> *(www.england.nhs.uk/about/equality)*

What are the components of culturally competent and virtuous leadership?

Halligan (2014) reminds us that:

> …if we always do what we've always done, we'll always get what we've always got. We don't need a randomised controlled trial to tell us what every healthcare worker knows – some wards, teams, departments, divisions and hospitals are better led than others and this perception goes well beyond able management or command. At its core, leadership is a purely moral and emotional activity. It is unconnected with seniority and only loosely related to intellect and it is about the ability to engage, motivate and inspire.

It is defined by our values and implies having moral courage, integrity and the conviction to accept accountability.

It could be argued that the pragmatism in Halligan's explanation of leadership was based on his vast experience as a clinician and medical educator, whilst the emphasis on virtues was influenced by Western and Eastern philosophers and leaders worldwide. Since this book is adopting an Aristotelian philosophical approach (although others have been acknowledged in the limited space provided; see Chapter 2), I will endeavour to provide the key components of what I have called 'culturally competent and virtuous leadership'.

A virtue, according to Aristotle, lies between two vices. For example, the virtue of courage lies between the vices of rashness and cowardice. The coward has too much fear, which leads to an inability to act or inappropriate action; the rash person has too little fear and excessive confidence, which may also lead to inappropriate or even harmful acts to the self and/or the person/purpose towards whom/which the courage is directed. The courageous person has the right amount of fear. Sellman (2011, p.40) explains that a virtuous act is an act in the right measure (the golden mean), although we should not suppose that a virtuous person will always hit the mean. However, even when the full virtue is not achieved, the efforts made towards it will be more likely to contribute to human flourishing than if no attempt was made at virtuous behaviour.

I propose that culturally competent and virtuous leadership lies between the vices of extreme collectivism and extreme self-interest/individualism. Leadership at either end of the leadership pole is toxic and can have catastrophic results, as many recent reports attest. Table 7.1 provides some suggestion of the toxic vices of leadership that may lie on the extreme ends of the leadership continuum.

Between the two toxic vices lie the components of culturally competent and virtuous leadership's golden mean, as depicted in Figure 7.1.

A culturally competent and virtuous leader is one who possesses deep self- awareness. An awareness of one's own cultural values and identity and the need for self-compassion is fundamental for a leader who wishes to inspire those she/he is working with. Crucial to this is the attainment of the virtue of proper self-love and to 'know thyself' (aftognosia), which guides our actions towards understanding, caring and respecting our self. It is important for

TABLE 7.1 The toxic vices of leadership.

Toxic effects of leadership based on extreme collectivism	*Toxic effects of leadership based on extreme self-interest/individualism*
- Co-dependence and co-collusion	- Self-interest-driven action
- Group think	- Lack of interest in each other as people
- Lack of whistle-blowers	- Exploitative behaviours
- In-group conformity pressure	- Competitiveness
- Exploitative, excessive interest in each other	- Lack of trust
- Lack of personal growth and low levels of self-awareness	- Lack of belongingness
- Lack of self-leadership	- Psychological insecurity
- Suppression of dissent and diverse opinions	- Destructive conflict
- Tolerance of poor standards of care	- Energy draining and burnout

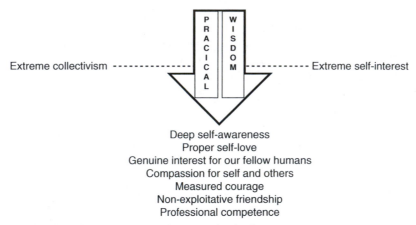

Extreme collectivism - Extreme self-interest

Deep self-awareness
Proper self-love
Genuine interest for our fellow humans
Compassion for self and others
Measured courage
Non-exploitative friendship
Professional competence

FIGURE 7.1   Culturally competent and virtuous leadership.

leaders to understand that their self is not complete without a relationship with the selves of those she/he leads and who may come from a variety of cultural backgrounds; therefore, equal amounts of culturally competent understanding, caring and respect must be given to them. The friendships of this leader are genuine channels of intercultural communication as well as enabling a connection with the person behind the professional worker.

In nurturing a virtuous working environment, this leader, through his/her own behaviour and culturally competent acts, is a compassionate role model who understands the emotional suffering of his/her co-workers and sensitively responds to them. Within this approach, leaders do not form friendships in order to exploit them for self-gain (such as self-advancement). Diversity is celebrated and the leader encourages staff to engage with it by providing co-learning opportunities. Openness and freedom to express views related to the improvement of the quality of services offered to patients is paramount. But even in such caring and democratic working environments, the enactment of measured courage is nurtured. Small- and medium-sized teams operate within larger organisations that continuously evolve to respond to changes to national policy, changes in the population, changes in science and technology, changes in the economy, changes in politics and so on. Not every change is consulted upon and not every change results in improvements. These are some of the factors that the culturally competent and virtuous leader considers seriously by asking:

- Are these the right changes, is this the right time for them and are they required for the right reasons?
- Do we have adequate understanding as to the effects of these changes on our work, and if not, what resources should I be providing for my team?
- How do I empower my team to have the courage to challenge changes that will not contribute to the flourishing of the patients, staff and organisation?
- What strategies should I be putting into place to help the team deal with the consequences of their speaking up?
- Am I able to provide culturally competent and compassionate support to my multicultural team when dealing with ethical dilemmas?

Apart from inspiring, supporting and empowering others, a leader is without a doubt the guardian of quality and standards. She/he has the responsibility, in collaboration with colleagues at different levels of the organisation, to promote high-quality service provision that is culturally and compassionately competent and strives to eliminate health inequalities. This means that the professional competences of all staff have to be kept updated and enhanced in order to cope with the ever-growing complexity of clinical practice in multicultural environments. Equally important is his/her contribution to nurturing high-quality working environments and championing employment standards that promote equal opportunities and human flourishing.

Leaders and leadership development

In the previous sections, I did not make any distinctions between leaders and leadership. However, some clarification about these two concepts will be beneficial.

West, et al. (2015), in discussing leadership development, suggest that leadership is a shared, collective process within organisations. Leaders are designated persons in positions of authority within the formal hierarchy of the organisation. However, West, et al. argue that the available research evidence highlights the importance of collective leadership and advocates for a balance between individual skill enhancement and organisational capacity building. A collective leadership culture is characterised by shared leadership where there is still a formal hierarchy, but power is dependent on who has the expertise at each moment. Research evidence suggests that shared leadership in teams predicts team effectiveness.

The same authors state that although organisational leadership development combining learning activities with practice activities has been recommended for the last decade, traditional leader-centric development programmes and a preoccupation with individual leader development have continued to dominate. Further, these authors advocate that collective leadership development depends on context and therefore it is likely to be best done 'in house' with expert support, highlighting the important contribution of organisation development and not just leader development. Evidence-based approaches to leadership development in healthcare are needed.

One such evidenced-based approach is that developed by a European-funded project that I coordinated during 2012–2014. Part of the Intercultural Education for Nurses in Europe (IENE) programme, the IENE4[2] project, produced a European model for developing culturally competent and compassionate leadership (http://ieneproject.eu). The following steps were implemented for the development of the model (http://ieneproject.eu/download/Outputs/IENE4%20%20European%20Model.pdf):

Step 1: Three integrative reviews of the literature on compassion were conducted.
Step 2: An online needs assessment of qualified nurses working in strategic-level and front-line services was administered in the seven participating countries.
Step 3: Two rounds of a Delphi study.
Step 4: A focus group.
Step 5: Implementation of the model to guide the development of two learning units by each project partner for the development of leadership at (a) the strategic level and (b) front-line service delivery.
Step 6: Piloting of the learning units in the seven participating countries.

Step 7:   Evaluation of the learning units by the pilot participants.

Step 8:   Learning units revised and finalised based on the evaluation feedback.

The model consists of four key constructs:

1.   Culturally Aware and Compassionate Healthcare Leadership (CACL)
2.   Culturally Knowledgeable and Compassionate Healthcare Leadership (CKCL)
3.   Culturally Sensitive and Compassionate Healthcare Leadership (CSCL)
4.   Culturally Competent and Compassionate Healthcare Leadership (CCCL)

Each key construct contains a map of statements – which were identified as priorities by the project's Delphi panel of experts – in the form of behaviours that the leaders need to develop in themselves and others in order to achieve the desired ethical organisational culture, as well as the leadership skills and qualities needed for virtuous, ethical decision-making and practice. For example, the construct of CACL contains the following statements:

1.1 Self-awareness as the first step for culturally competent compassionate leadership
1.2 Self-compassion as a necessity for culturally competent compassionate leadership
1.3 Acknowledgement of patients' and staff's diverse needs and responding to them with compassion
1.4 Cultivating and promoting moral virtues within the working environment
1.5 Doing the right thing for its own sake

Conclusion

The challenges of developing culturally competent and compassionate/virtuous leaders and leadership must not be underestimated. To ignore them would be a disastrous mistake, as ineffective leadership that lacks compassion can be dehumanising to patients and staff alike. This chapter has provided the reasons why leadership at all levels of an organisation should aim to be ethical, compassionate and culturally competent. As described in this chapter, new examples are emerging that are challenging the dominant models of twentieth-century leader development by introducing notions of collective leadership based on human virtues and ethics, as well as acknowledging the importance of cultural competence.

SUMMARY

- The complexities of multicultural societies and the growing health inequalities require that nursing and the health professions achieve culturally competent and virtuous leadership.
- Culturally competent and virtuous leadership is an ethical activity that is founded on virtues such as compassion, honesty, kindness, fairness, altruism and cooperation.
- Nursing must cultivate the virtue of practical wisdom (phronesis), as this is the virtue by which all other virtues (those of the intellect and of the character) are given appropriate expression.

- According to Aristotle (384–322 BCE), practical wisdom is the ability to do the right thing at the right time and for the right reasons.
- Non-virtuous leadership can be toxic for individuals and the collective.
- The IENE4 European model for culturally competent and compassionate leadership is introduced as an example of good practice.

LEARNING ACTIVITY

Access the report of the IENE4 leadership model and learning tools at http://ieneproject. eu/download/Outputs/Report_of_the_tools.PDF.

Browse through the report to discover how the leadership model was developed and validated and how the learning units associated with the model were developed and evaluated. Select the learning tool most relevant to your work from the ones included in the report. Read it and write a short reflective account on how informative and useful the tool was.

Notes

1 Transcultural nursing is caring that responds to the uniqueness of individuals in a culturally competent and compassionate way.
2 Strengthening Nurses' and Health Care Professionals' Capacity to Deliver Culturally Competent and Compassionate Care.

References

Aristotle (1989). *Rhetoric*. Cambridge, MA: Loeb Classic Library.

Aristotle (2004). *Nicomachean ethics*. Book II. London, UK: Penguin Classics.

Cook, R., Foglia, M.B., Landon, M.K., Melissa, M. and Bottrell, M.M. (2015). *Preventive ethics: Addressing ethics quality gaps on a systems level*. 2nd ed. Washington, DC: U.S. Department of Veterans Affairs; National Center for Ethics in Health Care.

Gallagher, A. (2006). The ethic of culturally competent health and social care. In: I. Papadopoulos, ed. *Transcultural health and social care: Development of culturally competent practitioners*. Edinburgh, UK: Churchill Livingstone Elsevier, pp. 65–84.

Gallagher, A. and Tschudin V. (2010). Educating for ethical leadership. *Nurse Education Today*, 30(3), pp. 224–227.

Goode, T.D. and Like, R.C. (2012). Advancing and sustaining cultural and linguistic competence in the American health system: Challenges, strategies, and lessons learned. In: D. Ingleby, A. Chiarenza, W. Deville and I. Kotsioni, eds. *Inequalities in health care for migrants and ethnic minorities*. Vol.2. COST series on health and diversity. Antwerp, The Netherlands: Garant Publishers, pp. 49–65.

Fox, E., Crigger, B., Bottrell, M. and Bauck, P., (nd). Ethical leadership: Fostering an ethical environment & culture. Retrieved from: www.ethics.va.gov/elprimer.pdf.

Francis, R. (2010). *The Mid Staffordshire NHS Foundation Trust Inquiry. The independent inquiry into care provided by Mid Staffordshire NHS Foundation Trust January 2005–March 2009*. London, UK: The Stationery Office.

Halligan, A. (2014). Learning leadership: How to become a leader in the NHS. Retrieved from: www. youtube.com/watch?v=d5ivSOstu3s.

King's Fund (2011). *The future of leadership and management in the NHS. No more heroes. Report from The King's Fund Commission on Leadership and Management in the NHS.* London, UK: King's Fund.

Papadopoulos, I., ed. (2006). *Transcultural health and social care: Development of culturally competent practitioners.* Edinburgh, UK: Churchill Livingstone Elsevier.

Sellman, D. (2011). *What makes a good nurse.* London, UK: Jessica Kingsley Publishers.

West, M., Armit, K., Loewenthal, L., Eckert, R., West, T. and Lee, A. (2015). *Leadership development in health care: The evidence base.* London, UK: The Faculty of Medical Leadership and Management with The King's Fund and the Center for Creative Leadership.

8

RESEARCHING CULTURALLY COMPETENT COMPASSION

LEARNING OBJECTIVES

Upon completion of this chapter, readers should be able to:

- Define culturally competent research and list its main characteristics.
- Discuss the innovative methods used to recruit and support volunteer researchers from different countries to co-develop an international online survey on culturally competent compassion in nursing.
- Discuss the benefits and limitations of collaborative international research and the production of knowledge and understanding related to culturally competent and compassionate nursing.

Introduction: the meaning of research

In 2006, I defined culturally competent research as an act that both utilises and develops knowledge and skills that promote the delivery of healthcare that is sensitive and appropriate to individuals' needs, whatever their cultural background (Papadopoulos, 2006b). I have also declared my support for the ideology of participatory research (PR), which focuses on people, power and praxis (Finn, 1994). PR is people-centred in the sense that the process of critical inquiry is informed by and responds to their experiences and needs. PR is about giving power to ordinary people. Power is crucial to the construction of reality, language, meanings and rituals of truth (Foucault, 1973). PR promotes empowerment through the development of common knowledge and critical awareness, which are suppressed by the dominant knowledge system. It is also about praxis (Lather, 1986; Maguire, 1987). It recognises the inseparability of theory and practice and critical awareness of the personal–political dialectic. It is grounded in an explicit political stance and a clearly articulated value base of social justice, as well as the transformation of those contemporary socio-cultural structures and processes that support the degeneration of participatory democracy, injustice and inequality.

The ideology of PR is very compatible with the aims of culturally competent research and topics such as culturally competent compassion. Democratising the production of knowledge through established and new methods and the involvement of people with and without research expertise at all levels of the research endeavour should be a desirable goal of anyone wishing to understand one of the most human of all emotions and behaviours – that of compassion. This chapter describes the research principles, methods and processes adopted during an international research collaboration on culturally competent compassion.

It is also a celebration and a wonderful example of what people from different cultures and countries can do when they work together with genuine interest. This collaboration and co-production is a testament to the compassion of this large group of people towards the nursing profession – and their fellow humans – that they have worked on this project with such enthusiasm and authenticity.

Researching culturally competent compassion

In 2014, stimulated by the public and scholarly debates about care without compassion, I decided to attempt an investigation into some of the issues around this topic that both the public and professionals appeared to agree upon.

I wanted to establish whether or not this topic interested nurses globally and whether or not there were similarities and differences with the issues that had emerged in the UK. To start with, I created a ten-question questionnaire that was piloted by seventy-three South Korean nurses.

People involvement and research volunteerism

In order to engage nurses from different countries, I emailed individuals belonging to my networks informing them of my project and requesting volunteers to join me in an exploration of the cultural similarities and differences of compassion in nursing. Within just an hour I had received over thirty expressions of interest. Respondents were a mixture of clinical nurses, nurse educators and some held practitioner–educator roles. Approximately half of them were known to me, whilst the other half were members of the same professional networks as myself but not known to me personally. I replied to all, giving them an outline of my intentions and how I envisaged their involvement in the project. My suggestion was to establish a short questionnaire survey and to administer this online. All individuals who expressed an interest were invited to join the project. In total, people from eighteen countries were recruited. At least two volunteer co-researchers formed each national team. If a participating country had only one volunteer co-researcher, a second person was recruited by the co-researcher in order to ensure that the workload was shared.

The following countries were originally involved:

1. Australia
2. Cyprus: (a) Greek Cypriots and (b) Turkish Cypriots
3. Colombia
4. Czech Republic
5. Greece

6. Hungary
7. Ireland
8. Italy
9. Israel
10. Japan
11. Norway
12. Philippines
13. Poland
14. Spain
15. Turkey
16. United Arab Emirates
17. United Kingdom
18. USA

Unfortunately, Ireland, Japan and the United Arab Emirates withdrew at the early stages, leaving fifteen participating countries with sixteen possible datasets. This situation arose because although Cyprus is one country, the current political situation meant that the two main ethnic groups were separately involved in the project.

Empowering the volunteer researchers

At the start of the collaboration, a set of notes, which functioned as an informal contract, was sent to all volunteer co-researchers in order to clarify the aim of the project, the contributions of everyone, the level of support available and the benefits to them and nursing. Box 8.1 provides an edited version of the document that was sent out.

To begin with, the original questionnaire was revised following its piloting in South Korea. The revised questionnaire was sent to all volunteer collaborators for comments, and once these were received, the questionnaire was adjusted and sent back to the national teams for translation and back-translation. Guidelines on how to deal with the translation were sent to everyone.

The main challenge that arose during the translation phase was the translation of the concept 'compassion'. A number of national teams reported that there was not one word that directly translated as 'compassion', and even when there was, its usage was a negative one (e.g. as 'pity'). Some teams had to consult colleagues regarding the 'best' word to choose out of a list of similar concepts. The questionnaire is now available in the following languages:

- Czech
- English
- Filipino
- Greek
- Hebrew
- Hungarian
- Italian
- Norwegian
- Polish
- Spanish
- Turkish

BOX 8.1 NOTES AND INSTRUCTIONS FOR THE VOLUNTEER RESEARCHERS

Exploring the cultural aspects of compassion in nursing

An international online survey

1. Purpose and research question
This ten-question on-line survey aims at a quick exploration of the following research question:

> Are there cultural differences in the way that compassion in nursing is understood and promoted?

The questionnaire has been piloted with nurses in South Korea.

2. My resources in the UK
I have been awarded a very small internal grant that will enable me to engage two early career members of staff to work on this project for a few hours per month for six months.

3. Your role
You all understand that this is an unpaid volunteer role that aims:

(a) To provide feedback on the draft questionnaire.
(b) To translate and back-translate the agreed questionnaire into the required language and to send the translated document to the coordinator to be processed.
(c) To administer the survey using your own nursing networks/connections and relevant nursing electronic lists you have accessed to. This online administration is the main method to be used. However, if for cultural or other reasons you wish to print and distribute the questionnaire, you may do so.
(d) To translate into English the comments that may be contained in the completed questionnaires.
(e) There are at least two volunteer researchers in each country. I recommend that you divide the workload. For example, one of you may do the translation whilst the other can do the back-translation, and so on.
f) To keep regular email communication with the UK coordinating team, responding to their queries as soon as you can.
g) To be involved in the analysis and writing of articles as little or as much as you wish or have time for.

4. Ethics permission
Although the UK coordinator will apply for ethics permission from the coordinating university, it is suggested that you check the guidelines of your institutions and, if required, apply and gain ethics permission from them.

5. Sample sizes

The 'ten-question' version of the survey on SurveyMonkey is *free*. However, it only allows up to 100 participants per country. In some of the larger countries we will have up to 100 people responding, whilst in others the number will be smaller. I suggest that the minimum you should aim for is fifty respondents from each country. But I recommend that we keep the survey open even when we reach the magical figure of fifty, as this stage will vary in time for each country.

6. Intellectual property (IP) and benefits

We will have a very generous approach to IP. We will all put much effort into this project, so we will all have equal access to the data. However, to avoid confusion, misunderstandings and possible chaos, I will have the overall IP as the originator, coordinator and principal investigator. All data will be stored at the coordinating university. Each country can store its own data (where there is more than one person in a country, an agreement has to be reached and I must be notified of the agreed arrangements).

I foresee the production of at least two articles authored by all. Co-researchers from participating countries may wish to author country-specific articles.

Any presentations that partners wish to make in their own countries or at international conferences must credit the work of the 'team' (everyone involved).

The outputs from this project will add to the growing body of knowledge about compassion in nursing, particularly the pioneering work of the coordinator who is the originator of culturally competent compassion.

7. Original Timetable

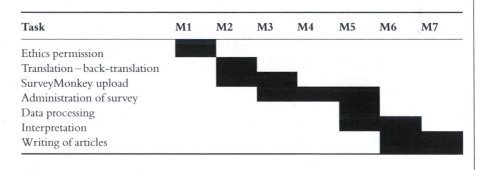

Task	M1	M2	M3	M4	M5	M6	M7
Ethics permission							
Translation – back–translation							
SurveyMonkey upload							
Administration of survey							
Data processing							
Interpretation							
Writing of articles							

The translated questionnaire was uploaded on the SurveyMonkey® software by the UK team. The link to each survey was sent to each national team along with the text of a standard explanation to accompany the survey that was used by all (after being translated if needed) as the front page of the survey.

The international online compassion questionnaire

The survey aimed to collect, in a short period of time, baseline data about various issues related to compassion in nursing that were being talked and written about. Although most of the questions were designed to be answered quickly by busy professionals, we also wanted to capture some explanations and provide the opportunity for participants to add their narratives. Therefore, Questions 1, 5 and 10a, asked for qualitative information.

1. How would you define the term 'compassion'?
   (a) Empathy and kindness
   (b) Deep awareness of the suffering of others
   (c) Deep awareness of the suffering of others and a wish to alleviate it
   (d) Other (please specify below)
2. How important is compassion in nursing?
   (a) Not very important
   (b) Important
   (c) Very important
3. Do you believe that compassion can be taught to nurses?
   (a) Yes
   (b) No
   (c) Don't know
4. Do you believe that compassion is being taught to nurses?
   (a) The correct amount and level of teaching is provided
   (b) Some teaching is provided
   (c) Not enough teaching is provided
   (d) Don't know
5. How is compassion demonstrated in practice? Please give examples.
6. Do you think patients prefer to be nursed by:
   (a) Knowledgeable nurses with good interpersonal skills?
   (b) Knowledgeable nurses with good technical skills?
   (c) Knowledgeable nurses with good management skills?
7. In your view, which is the most important influence for developing compassion?
   (a) The person's family
   (b) The person's cultural values
   (c) The person's personal experience of compassion
8. Please select the statement you most agree with
   (a) [Country's name] patients value efficiency more than compassion
   (b) [Country's name] patients value the use of medical technology more than the use of compassion
   (c) [Country's name] patients value medical treatment more than compassionate caring
9. Please select the statement you most agree with
   (a) Nurses in [country] experience compassion from their managers
   (b) Nurses in [country] experience compassion from their colleagues
   (c) Nurses in [country] experience compassion from their patients
10. Please select the option which applies to you
   (a) I am a final-year student nurse
   (b) I am a qualified practising nurse
   (c) I am a nurse educator

TABLE 8.1 Sample sizes and countries of participants' residence.

Country of residence and work of participants	Number of respondents
Australia	35
Colombia	103
Cyprus	
Greek Cypriots	49
Turkish Cypriots	73
Czech Republic	142
Greece	94
Hungary	87
Israel	81
Italy	53
Norway	29
Philippines	100
Poland	101
Spain	174
Turkey	96
United Kingdom	56
United States of America	50
Total	1323

10a. Finally, please
- (a) State your ethnic origin
- (b) Offer any comments, advice, views or stories that can shed light on the meaning and use of compassion by [country] nurses

The response to the survey

A total of 1323 nurses from fifteen countries completed the compassion survey.

The breakdown of responses per country is shown in Table 8.1.

The survey generated a large dataset of quantitative and qualitative data. Each country's responses to the open-ended questions were sent to the respective co-researchers for translation and for quality checks of accuracy and meaning. The national teams were asked to provide the first-level analysis, which consisted of the key issues that were identified whilst reading and translating the data. All translated data were sent to the UK team for in-depth country and comparative analysis.

Data analysis

Qualitative analysis

The data were imported into the NVivo software. Thematic analysis (Braun and Clarke, 2006) was used. One researcher coded the text piece by piece with initial descriptive codes. The codes were then grouped into themes and a coding manual was developed. The codes and themes were discussed by the UK research coordinating team. Any disagreements were discussed and resolved. Each country was sent the analysis of their own data for verification.

Quantitative data

Data were entered into SPSS and a descriptive analysis was undertaken. The results of this analysis were sent to all countries. Inferential analysis was also conducted and a structural equation modelling approach was used in order to investigate whether responses to one question would predict the response to another question on the survey.

Both qualitative and quantitative data of all countries were aggregated together as well as compared between countries.

Summary of findings

Definition of compassion

The majority of participants defined compassion as a deep awareness of the suffering of others and a wish to alleviate it. Other definitions worth reporting here were:

- Being able to see the others as equal and include them with respect in their sadness, their joy, their adversity or their walk through life, never from a moralistic perspective, but with an attitude of solidarity (Colombian participant)
- Good and equal care (Turkish Cypriot participant)
- Empathy in the spirit of following the emotions of the other person, effort to connect to the person and effort to find together a path to mitigate the problems of his or her suffering (Czech Republic participant)

The analysis revealed that participants considered compassion as a conscious and intentional act consisting of a complex list of components and actions (Papadopoulos, et al., 2017). These are shown in Figure 8.1.

Time

Nurses reported making conscious efforts to overcome the constraints of time. An Australian participant stated that making patients feel that their suffering is worthy of the nurses' time is very important, whilst a Greek nurse expressed the view that compassion is about devoting time to be with the patients and simply holding their hand when they are in pain.

Being there

An American nurse explained that recognising the important times for the patient and being there for them is crucial and comforting. A nurse from the Czech Republic described a similar sentiment, stating that nurses should be able to express compassion in the moment.

Going the extra mile

Giving extra time to a lonely patient, doing acts of benevolence that go beyond one's job and making a phone call to ask about the transition from hospital to home were examples given by Italian, Norwegian, Spanish and Colombians participants, some of whom also suggested that

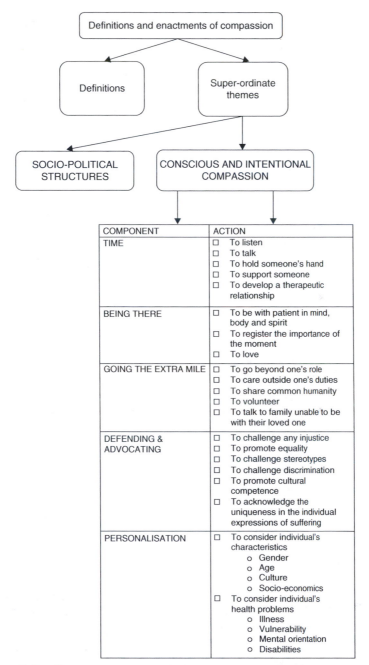

FIGURE 8.1 Culturally competent compassion – components and actions.

Source: 'Exploring nurses' meaning and experiences of compassion: an international online survey involving 15 countries. 2017. Used with permission. (*Journal of Transcultural Nursing*, 28, pp. 286–295.)

maybe some of these acts by nurses are done not because they are part of their job but because they are compassionate human beings.

Defending and advocating

Many participants stated that protecting the human rights of vulnerable people was central to compassionate practice. A participant from Turkey suggested that nurses listen to patients and their families, actively trying to understand their problems, pain, anger or love in order to help them.

Personalisation

A participant from Israel wrote that nurses should understand that each person's suffering is subjective and unique, whilst a participant from Philippines stated that compassion requires cultural awareness.

Learning to be a compassionate nurse

The majority of the participants (97%) declared that compassion is important in nursing. Nearly 60% believed that compassion can be taught to nurses, whilst a quarter (25%) of the participants did not believe that it can. However, only 11% of the participants reported that the correct amount of compassion content was being taught, with a much larger percentage reporting that not enough was being taught (44%). In terms of important influences in developing compassion, the participants were almost equally divided between the following three influences: the family, individual cultural values and personal experiences of compassion.

Receiving compassion at work

Almost 50% of the participants reported that that they receive compassion from patients. A further 46% reported receiving compassion from colleagues. Sadly, only 4% reported receiving compassion from their managers. This significant finding was reported by all participants with the exception of those from Philippines and the Turkish-speaking Cypriots.

The influence of socio-political structures on compassion and care

The data revealed the impact of socio-political influences on perceptions of compassion and the conscious and intentional nature of compassion. Nearly every piece of data had a policy or political dimension that illustrated the differences in health service provision, status and power of nursing in the participating countries. Nurses felt constrained and influenced by socio-political structural issues that affected the delivery of care. Such structures determine the context in which healthcare is provided and thus the macro-environment in which nurses practise. Decisions about the funding of and access to healthcare can have ramifications beyond healthcare services, affecting wider society and societal relationships. Our participants appeared to be acutely aware of the influences of socio-political decisions on their actions.

While there are differences in the way healthcare is delivered between the countries surveyed in this study (e.g. in terms of degrees of poverty, stability and levels of coverage of healthcare), our participants demonstrated many similarities in terms of their roles in relation to the provision of compassionate care. And while there was similarity across countries in terms of feeling that compassionate care can be constrained by policies that aimed to contain the costs of delivering health services, there were some differences between countries in relation to actions and reactions to these perceived constraints. Aspects of the policy, infrastructure and societal struggles that influence perceptions of compassion were evident (e.g. target-driven policies in the UK, legacy of a lack of universal coverage in the USA, conflict in Colombia and austerity measures in Greece).

In conclusion, the findings suggest that one's country of residence, cultural background, personal experiences and the context of one's work influence the way one defines compassion. The findings clearly indicate the need for culturally competent compassion within the education programmes of nurses.

A more extensive report of the qualitative and quantitative data from this study can be found in two published articles (Papadopoulos, et al., 2016a, 2017).

Reflections of a coordinator

Venturing into international research with only a 'few pennies' for a budget requires a lot of courage and passion! But when the topic of research is one that people from around the world believe in as passionately as you do and it is not only relevant but very important to nursing, the task at hand becomes easier. So, we are halfway towards achieving the goal of Principle 1 of PR (people). Taking the time to consult all of those people who volunteered to work on the project, even though many had little research experience, is also part of Principle 1.

Listening with cultural sensitivity to people's views, ideas, experiences and needs straddles Principles 1 and 2 (power), in my view. Providing clear instructions, regular communications and relevant information to co-researchers, as well as supporting them in tasks that they may not have time to do or they may find difficult, can be very empowering, especially if this is done in a respectful way, even by someone you have never met in person. Successful collaborations are those that include people with complementary skills. Successful collaborations also nurture goodwill and compassion for the collective through personal growth opportunities that enable persons to bring about change for the common good. This is how Principle 2 can be achieved!

As the coordinator of this project, I tried my best to adhere to Principle 3: praxis. I hope very much that my co-researchers found me to be fair and democratic, although I am aware that sometimes, for practical reasons, I took decisions without full consultation. I believe that this happens of necessity when time, resources and the sheer scale of the operation may not allow the implementation of the ideal practice. However, when there is trust and openness, there should not be fear in treading the path towards the agreed goal.

Engaging in the production of knowledge is incredibly political. In particular, knowledge that is derived from the bottom up can be more powerful than that which is driven from the top down. Bottom-up knowledge has people power behind it, which can be a powerful, lasting force that can achieve the positive transformation that people need and want. The articles that are based on the data from this research project can bring about transformation in processes and structures. However, it is worth remembering the wise words of the Greek philosopher, Aristotle, who asserted that "What lies in our power to do, also lies in our power not to do."

LEARNING ACTIVITY

The consortium working on the international online compassion survey published the following two articles:

- Papadopoulos, I., Taylor, G., Ali, S., Aagard, M., Akman, O., Alpers, L.M., …, Zorba, A. (2017). Exploring nurses' meaning and experiences of compassion: An international online survey involving 15 countries. *Journal of Transcultural Nursing*, 28, pp. 286–295.
- Papadopoulos, I., Zorba, A., Koulouglioti, C., Ali, S., Aagard, M., Akman, O., …, Vasiliou, M. (2016). International study on nurses' views and experiences of compassion. *International Nursing Review*, 63, pp. 395–405.

The first presents the analysis of the qualitative data, whilst the second presents the analysis of the quantitative data. Ideally, it would be beneficial if you could read both articles, but if your time is limited, please choose one of them. Read the article and write a review about it, concentrating on what aspects you found interesting and useful to your work. You may wish to send your review to the journal who published the article and request that this is published, or you may discuss the article and your review of it at your journal club or team meeting.

References

Braun, V. and Clarke, V. (2006). Using thematic analysis in psychology. *Qualitative Research in Psychology*, 3, pp. 77–101.

Finn, J. (1994). The promise of participatory research. *Journal of Progressive Human Services*, 5(2), pp. 25–42.

Foucault, M. (1973). *The order of things: An archaeology of the human science*. New York, NY: Vintage Books.

Lather, P. (1986). Research as praxis. *Harvard Educational Review*, 56(3), pp. 257–277.

Maguire, P. (1987). *Doing participatory research: A feminist approach*. Amherst, MA: University of Massachusetts.

Papadopoulos, I. (2006a). Developing culturally competent researchers: A model for its development. In: J. Nazroo, ed. *Health and social research in multiethnic societies*. London, UK: Routledge, pp. 82–94.

Papadopoulos, I. (2006b). Culturally competent research. In: I. Papadopoulos, ed. *Transcultural health and social care: Development of culturally competent practitioners*. Edinburgh, UK: Churchill Livingstone Elsevier, pp. 85–98.

Papadopoulos, I., Kouta, C., Malliarou, M., Shea, S., Apostolara, P. and Vasiliou, M. (2016b). Exploring the cultural aspects of compassion in nursing care: A comparative study of Greece and Cyprus. *International Journal of Caring Sciences*, 9, pp. 471–480.

Papadopoulos, I., Taylor, G., Ali, S., Aagard, M., Akman, O., Alpers, L.M., …, Zorba, A. (2017). Exploring nurses meaning and experiences of compassion: an international online survey involving 15 countries. *Journal of Transcultural Nursing*, 28, pp. 286–295.

Papadopoulos, I., Zorba, A., Koulouglioti, C., Ali, S., Aagard, M., Akman, O., …, Vasiliou, M. (2016a). International study on nurses' views and experiences of compassion. *International Nursing Review*, 63, pp. 395–405.

9

MEASURING COMPASSION

LEARNING OBJECTIVES

Upon completion of this chapter, readers should be able to:

- Discuss why compassion should be measured and the opposition that has been raised about this development.
- Discuss the methodological steps and approaches taken in the development of the Papadopoulos/IENE4 self-assessment tool of cultural and compassionate competence.
- Specifically describe how the tool's content validity and reliability were achieved.
- Visit the open access http://ieneproject.eu/assessment.php, complete their online assessment and obtain their level of cultural and compassionate competence.

Introduction

Why we need to measure compassion in practice?

Bradshaw (2009) writes that, in the UK, the Secretary of State for Health announced in 2008 that the quality of compassion within the NHS was to be measured. This was probably a reaction to a Healthcare Commission (2007) report on complaints about the NHS in England that was published at the time, which reported that 7% of the complaints referred to nursing issues and attitudes. The Secretary of State for Health (Johnson, 2008) stated that patients had the right to be treated with dignity, respect and compassion and asserted that measuring such factors will ensure that the quality of care is improved.

The intention of the NHS to measure compassion was met with both approval and disapproval within the nursing profession. Bradshaw (2009) reported that the Royal College of Nursing was very supportive, whilst Mooney (2009) quoted Professor Peter Griffiths, director of the then National Nursing Research Unit, who, whilst declaring his support to the proposal, stated that measuring human compassion is hugely challenging. She also quoted Lesley Baillie, a principal lecturer at Southbank University, who opposed the proposal by asking:

> How do you measure a light touch, silence or an important phone call? It is situation and individual specific. There is a risk if you try to turn compassion into a check list, it will become less than it really is, and how meaningful is that?

Others objected to individual compassion being measured, as this could lead to accusations that some individuals are not sufficiently compassionate and consequently being blamed for failings that related to external factors such as a lack of resources, organisational management or restructuring (Crawford, et al., 2014).

Despite the government's intentions and the intense debate in the mass and social media at the time, to date, the NHS has not funded nor adopted a reliable and validated measuring tool to measure individual compassion. Some clinical nursing leaders as well as some universities have reported using methods to assess individuals' compassion at the recruitment stage. However, numerous studies have reported that the disposition to compassion the students have at the early stages of their training diminishes over time, especially once they are immersed into clinical practice (Hojat, et al., 2009; Neumann, et al., 2011). This indicates the need to ensure that both the theoretical and practical components of nursing curricula nurture the development of compassion, a topic that is addressed in Chapter 6.

Another reason why compassion needs to be measured is the accumulation of evidence that compassion is associated with positive clinician outcomes such as job satisfaction, as well as patient satisfaction, compliance and motivation (van der Cingel, 2011; Way and Tracy, 2012). Safeguarding reasons also require that both individual and organisational levels of compassion are measured to ensure that incidents of care void of compassion (The Patients Association, 2009; Francis 2010, 2013; Abraham, 2011; Cummings and Bennett, 2012) and its disastrous impacts on often vulnerable human beings are eliminated.

How can measuring tools be used to enhance patient care?

Strauss, et al. (2016) conducted a review of the literature in order to identify definitions and measures of compassion. Their rationale was that despite the increasing recognition of the importance of compassion, there is a lack of consensus on its definition and a paucity of psychometrically robust measures for it. Their review yielded five elements of compassion that they suggested can be used to create robust measuring tools. The five elements are: recognising suffering; understanding the universality of human suffering; feeling for the person suffering; tolerating uncomfortable feelings; and motivation to act/acting to alleviate suffering. They argued that the absence of an acceptable definition has impeded scientific enquiry, with negative ramifications on research, education and practice. The review assumed that compassion could indeed be measured with questionnaire tools and that individual levels of compassion should be measured, but acknowledged the views of those who raised concerns about what should be measured and how (Dewar, et al., 2011). Strauss and her colleagues suggested that, as with many psychological variables, questionnaire measures may only provide a partial picture of compassion. They expressed the view that well-designed and reliable tools that acknowledge the complexities around measuring compassion have the potential to identify educational and practice-related interventions, both at an individual and an organisational level, which will enhance self-compassion and the compassion provided to patients, colleagues and others.

Tools for measuring culturally competent compassion

Two years before Strauss and her colleagues published their review of the literature on the definition and measures of compassion, a colleague and I conducted an integrative review of the literature on tools for measuring culturally competent compassion. Notwithstanding national and international pronouncements about the importance of compassion, which have been discussed in previous chapters, our motivation for the review was based on the requirement by the British Nursing and Midwifery Council (NMC) for care to be compassionate and non-discriminatory and to value diversity, as well as the belief that compassion not only was enacted differently by the populations of different cultural groups, but was also inadequately measured in practice.

Sadly the literature searches failed to yield any articles that addressed 'culturally competent compassion'. Nevertheless, we proceeded to conduct a review on how 'compassion' is being measured in nursing and in other healthcare professions (Papadopoulos and Ali, 2015). Of the 1683 articles initially identified, only 305 appeared to meet the inclusion criteria based on their abstracts. After further screening, only six research articles qualified for inclusion in the review (Box 9.1). This reflects the dearth of empirical literature on measuring compassion and highlights the need for further research on this subject.

BOX 9.1 THE SIX STUDIES OF THE INTEGRATIVE REVIEW OF THE LITERATURE ON MEASURING COMPASSION

- Burnell, L. and Agan, D. (2013). Compassionate care: Can it be defined and measured? The development of the Compassionate Care Assessment Tool. *International Journal of Caring Sciences*, 6(2), pp. 180–187.
- Dewar, B., Pullin, S. and Tocheris, R. (2011). Valuing compassion through definition and measurement. *Nursing Management*, 17(8), pp. 32–37.
- Dhawan, N., Steinbach, A.B. and Halpern, J. (2007). Physician empathy and compassion for inmate-patients in the correctional health care setting. *Journal of Correctional Health Care*, 13(4), pp. 257–267.
- Fogarty, L.A., Curbow, B.A., Wingard, J.R., McDonnell, K. and Somerfield, M.R. (1999). Can 40 seconds of compassion reduce patient anxiety? *Journal of Clinical Oncology*, 17(1), pp. 371–379.
- Kret, D. (2011). The qualities of a compassionate nurse according to the perceptions of medical-surgical patients. *Medsurg Nursing*, 20(1), pp. 29–36.
- Roberts, L.W., Warner, T.D., Moutier, C., Geppert, C.M.A. and Hammond, K.A.G. (2011). Are doctors who have been ill more compassionate? Attitudes of resident physicians regarding personal health issues and the expression of compassion in clinical care. *Psychosomatics*, 52, pp. 367–374.

From these articles, we extracted data about each study's characteristics, such as the country where the study was conducted, the aim of the study, the design, the sample type and size, instruments used and conclusions.

The quality of the included studies was varied. For the majority of them, the stimuli and procedures were well-described, but one of the studies (Dewar, Pullin and Tocheris, 2011) did not provide enough description in order for the study to be replicated.

Most of the studies described how the participants were recruited and how informed consent was obtained. Sample sizes ranged from 78 to 250 participants. However, two of the studies had a low number of responses compared to the number of people who were initially invited to the study (Dhawan, et al., 2007; Fogarty, et al., 1999). This limits the validity of the findings and may have introduced selection bias. Moreover, one study (Dewar, Pullin and Tocheris, 2011) did not report the sample size.

Compassion was defined and operationalised differently in the included studies. This heterogeneity of the definitions of compassion made it difficult to compare the studies and assess the face validity of these measures.

Of the measures that were identified in our review, the compassionate care assessment tool (Burnell and Agan, 2013) appeared to be the most comprehensive. However, this measure has only been validated with inpatients, and it is not clear whether it can be adapted for use by other groups of patients, healthcare professionals (to rate their own compassion) or managers (to rate the compassion of healthcare professionals). Fogarty, et al.'s (1999) compassion rating scale has been validated both in physicians and nurses and has been used by patients to rate the compassion of their care provider. However, this scale is brief and limited in the scope of the different aspects of compassion that are being measured. Therefore, on the basis of this review, we cannot exclusively recommend one of these measures of compassion, a conclusion that is in line with that of Strauss, et al. (2016), who suggested that existing measures of compassion are not comprehensive enough and lacking in sufficient quality to measure all aspects of compassion.

The IENE4 project: Developing a measuring tool

The previous chapters provided ample evidence that healthcare should be administered not only with compassion, but also in a culturally competent manner, taking into account the values, culture and health beliefs of the individual. Culturally competent compassion may be defined as "the human quality of understanding the suffering of others and wanting to do something about it using culturally appropriate and acceptable caring interventions" (Papadopoulos, 2011).

The IENE4 project (http://ieneproject.eu/assessment.php) sought to develop an online self-assessment measuring tool that can be completed by nurses and other healthcare professionals in order to assess their own levels of culturally competent compassion and to improve upon them if needed (Papadopoulos, Ali and le Boutillier, forthcoming).

Developing the statements for the measuring tool

Drawing from the literature review outlined above and two others that were conducted as part of the IENE4 project (Petersen, et al., 2015), a number of statements in relation to culturally

TABLE 9.1 Number of statements in initial version of the tool.

Heading	Number of items
Universal/generic	
Cultural awareness	21
Cultural knowledge	12
Cultural sensitivity	16
Cultural competence	17
Client group-specific	
Mental health	5
Physical health	5
Older people	26
Children	14
Total	**116**

competent compassion in healthcare were compiled. Statements were also adapted from items included in an existing validated tool for measuring cultural competence (Papadopoulos, Tilki and Lees, 2004). The statements aimed to capture several aspects of compassion and cultural competence, including universal elements of compassion and culture-specific aspects of compassion. The tool also aimed to include statements that would be specific to healthcare professionals' working contexts and particular client groups.

A total of 116 statements were initially generated and these were grouped under specific headings (Table 9.1). The universal/generic statements were grouped using the framework of the Papadopoulos model of culturally competent compassion (Papadopoulos, 2014), which includes four constructs: culturally aware compassion, culturally knowledgeable compassion, culturally sensitive compassion and culturally competent compassion.

The client group-specific statements were grouped into: (a) mental health, (b) physical health, (c) older people and (d) children to enable the production of the four variations of the measuring tool.

The Delphi studies and content validity

The Delphi technique was used as a method for ensuring face and content validity of the measuring tool. The Delphi technique is a research method in which the opinions of a panel of experts are used to reach a consensus about a particular topic of concern (McKenna, 1994). Individuals from clinical practice and academia were invited to be part of the Delphi panel if they had expertise in one or more of the following topics: compassion, nursing or cultural competence. Each of the IENE4 partner institutions (the UK, Cyprus, Denmark, Spain, Romania, Italy and Turkey) recruited two experts to the panel; thus, there were fourteen Delphi members in total.

Two rounds of Delphi were undertaken. The responses of the first Delphi panel were analysed for central tendency and variability, and the mean, standard deviation, range, median and mode were assessed. Judgements were made based on these values and the recommendations of the Delphi panel as to which statements should be kept and which should be removed from the tool.

Mean rankings of the statements were analysed. A high ranking (low numerical value) of a statement was an indicator that the statement had a greater degree of relevance. Any statements that received very high median or mode values (indicating a low ranking) relative to other statements were considered for removal and most of them were removed from the tool. The aim was to include the items with the highest relevance (shown by high rankings), but also to include measures that covered all aspects of compassion and cultural competence. Decisions about removal of statements were discussed between the project team.

In the second round of the Delphi study, the four different versions of the tool were created, as discussed above. Delphi members were asked to complete all four versions of the tool by indicating whether they agreed or disagreed with each statement on a four-point scale (strongly agree, agree, disagree and strongly disagree).

Refining and updating the tool

Following the second round of the Delphi exercise, the project team examined the responses to the statements and the extent to which the Delphi members agreed or disagreed with the statements. If the Delphi panel advised that any statements should be removed, these were removed. The responses from some of the Delphi panel indicated that a few of the statements may be misinterpreted due to the use of negation and recommended their grammatical structure was changed to avoid this; their advice was implemented.

The four tools were compared against each other to ensure that each contained a similar number of statements in each of the four sections of the tool (awareness, knowledge, sensitivity and competence) and that each tool had a similar number of universal and client-specific statements.

The final tools consisted of: (a) the children's tool: thirty-three statements; (b) the adult mental health tool: thirty-four statements; (c) the older people tool: thirty-two statements; and (d) the adult physical health tool: thirty-three statements.

Guided by the Papadopoulos model (2014) for developing culturally competent and compassionate healthcare professionals, the statements under the cultural awareness heading were related to both self-compassion and the healthcare professionals' understanding of universal aspects of compassion. They included statements such as "I seek support from colleagues in order to process the emotional burden of my job," and "People in some cultures ignore and suppress their personal suffering and pretend it does not exist." Items under the cultural knowledge heading were related to the healthcare professionals' knowledge of the similarities and differences between cultures in terms of the way that compassion is understood; for example, "I recognise that some patients' beliefs may differ from my own but I can disagree with them in a respectful manner." The cultural sensitivity heading included items relating to giving compassion to and receiving compassion from patients and forming culturally appropriate and compassionate therapeutic relationships. This included statements such as, "Caring conversations and emotional connection with the patients are essential for compassionate care." Finally, the cultural competence heading related to the practice of compassion despite potential barriers. It included the item: "Compassion compels me to not only acknowledge, but also to act towards alleviating the suffering and pain of others."

Each tool also included questions in relation to the participants' demographic details and an open-ended question in which the participant could provide comments about their experience of using the tool and suggestions for any improvements. The four versions of the tool were translated from English into Spanish, Danish, Romanian, Turkish, Greek and Italian to enable participants to complete the tool in their country's native language. The quality of the translations was ensured through back-translation. All tools are now available in open access on the IENE website (http://ieneproject.eu/assessment.php).

Piloting the tool

The tool (in its four variations) was piloted with a large sample (n = 768) of healthcare professionals from the seven participating countries. The data were collected from June to September 2015.

Participants were eligible to take part in the study if they were qualified health professionals, final-year nursing students or practitioners and their job involved working with any one of the patient groups for which variations of the measuring tool was produced: (a) children, (b) older adults, (c) adult mental health and (d) adult physical health.

Participants were recruited via snowball and convenience sampling. Data was collected using an online survey software (Qualtrics, 2015). Participants completed and submitted the tool online.

Reliability testing

Statistical analyses were conducted using SPSS statistical software version 21 (IBM Corp., 2012). A reliability analysis was performed and initial analyses established the overall internal consistency of each of the four tools using Cronbach's alpha. The SPSS 'scale if item deleted' procedure was used in order to examine whether removing an item from the scale would improve its reliability.

This was followed by an assessment of each statement in each of the four sections of the tool, where chi-square analyses and analyses of description and frequency were conducted.

We aimed to assess the agreement between what we deemed to be the correct answer and the actual responses that the participants gave. In order to achieve this, the data were recoded from a four-point Likert score (1 to 4) into a dichotomous incorrect/correct variable (0 or 1). Therefore, each item was given a score of either 1 (correct) or 0 (incorrect). For most of the items, a response of 3 (agree) or 4 (strongly agree) was regarded as the 'correct' response and this was given a score of 1. A response of 1 (strongly disagree) or 2 (disagree) was considered 'incorrect' and therefore given a score of 0. For the reversed items, a response of 1 or 2 was considered correct and was given a score of 1, whereas a response of 3 or 4 was considered incorrect and given a score of 0. One-way chi-square analyses were conducted using these dichotomous data for each single item in turn to assess the difference between observed and expected results.

Results

The demographics of the sample (n = 768) are shown in Table 9.2 separated by specialism (adult mental health, children, older adults and adult physical health). The majority of participants were female and in the age range of twenty-one to fifty years. In terms of job role, the sample consisted of nurses and other health professionals, such as psychologists, physiotherapists, healthcare assistants and pharmacists.

TABLE 9.2 Demographics of the sample.

	Adult mental health	Children	Older adults	Adult physical health
Gender				
Male	35	24	38	32
Female	121	153	150	157
Not stated	6	24	16	12
Age				
Under 21	1	3	2	2
21–35	83	86	95	84
36–50	51	66	71	74
51–65	21	22	19	29
Over 65	0	0	1	0
Not stated	6	24	1	12

TABLE 9.3 Reliability of the four tools.

Measure	Cronbach's alpha
Children	0.78
Mental health	0.80
Older adults	0.77
Physical health	0.86

Reliability

The assessment of internal consistency showed that the four tools were very reliable. For each tool, the 'if-item-removed' analyses showed that all of the items contributed to the overall measure and none of the items needed to be removed. As can be seen in Table 9.3, all four versions of the tool had a Cronbach's alpha score higher than 0.7, which demonstrated a good level of reliability.

Chi-square analysis was used to measure the level of agreement between what we deemed to be the correct answers for the tool and the actual responses of the participants completing the tool. This was tested against a null hypothesis that all cells would yield equal responses. Descriptive analyses were also carried out in order to examine the responses of the participants to each of the items (e.g. the percentage of correct and incorrect responses for each item).

Overall, the results showed that the majority of items on the tool yielded proportionately more correct than incorrect responses and that there was a high level of agreement between the correct response and the responses that were actually observed in the study. This indicated that culturally competent compassion was being reliably measured by the four tools.

The final versions of the tool

As mentioned previously, a dichotomous scoring method was used whereby a correct answer received a score of 1 and an incorrect answer received a score of 0. The scores for all of the items are summed together to obtain a total score for culturally competent compassion. When calculating a total score for culturally competent compassion, the points from the four domains are counted equally. Therefore, a total score is calculated by adding together the scores from each of the four domains (culturally aware compassion, culturally knowledgeable compassion, culturally sensitive compassion and culturally competent compassion).

Depending on their score, a person completing this tool can achieve one of four possible levels of culturally competent compassion: incompetent, aware, safe or competent.

The final tools were uploaded onto the IENE project's website, which is a resource for the education of health professionals. The tools have been translated into Italian, Spanish, Danish, Turkish, Greek and Romanian and can currently be completed online by healthcare workers (at http://ieneproject.eu/assessment.php). Upon completion of a tool, the score is immediately provided, along with relevant feedback regarding what the score means and advice on how to improve it.

Conclusion

The evidence provided in this chapter as well as other chapters in this book show that urgent attention needs to be given to improving the levels of compassion afforded to patients, especially those who are most vulnerable, such as older people, people with mental health problems and children. In order to ensure this improvement occurs, easy-to-use validated and reliable tools that enable nurses and other health professionals to learn how to provide care with compassion must be developed and used. It is imperative that such tools recognise the multicultural nature of societies and promote the notion that humans understand and enact compassion in different ways depending on their culture. But this is not enough. Healthcare education and practice must stop avoiding the measuring of compassion. Although compassion is a complex and often subjective notion, researchers, academics, practitioners and patients should collaborate in order to find creative and innovative ways of measuring it. The evidence provided in the growing literature, some of which was discussed in this chapter, attests to the fact that compassion can be taught, assessed and measured.

This chapter has presented the details of developing the Papadopoulos/IENE tool that measures the level of cultural and compassionate competence of healthcare practitioners. This reliable and valid tool is the first of its kind and it is available in open access in several languages and can be self-administered online by anyone who wishes to find out how culturally and compassionately competent they are.

LEARNING ACTIVITY

Assess yourself using the Papadopoulos/IENE4 measuring tool. Go to http://ieneproject. eu/assessment.php and learn your level of competence and what you need to do in order to improve it.

References

Abraham, A. (2011). Care and compassion? Report of the Health Service Ombudsman on ten investigations into NHS care of older people. Retrieved January 2018 from: www.gov.uk/government/publications/report-of-the-health-service-ombudsman-on-ten-investigations-into-nhs-care-of-older-people.

Bradshaw, A. (2009). Measuring nursing care and compassion: The McDonalised nurse? *Journal of Medical Ethics*, 35, pp. 465–468.

Burnell, L. and Agan, D.L. (2013). Compassionate care: Can it be defined and measured? The development of the compassionate care assessment tool. *International Journal of Caring Sciences*, 6, pp. 180–187.

Crawford, P., Brown, B., Kvangarsnes, M. and Gilbert, P. (2014). The design of compassionate care. *Journal of Clinical Nursing*, 23, pp. 3589–3599.

Cummings, J. and Bennett, V. (2012). Developing the culture of compassionate care. Creating a new vision for nurses, midwives and care-givers. NHS Commissioning Board. Retrieved January 2018 from: www.england.nhs.uk/wp-content/uploads/2012/12/compassion-in-practice.pdf.

Dewar, B., Pullin, S. and Tocheris, R. (2011). Valuing compassion through definition and measurement. *Nursing Management*, 17(9), pp. 32–37.

Dhawan, N., Steinbach, A.B. and Halpern, J. (2007). Physician empathy and compassion for inmate-patients in the correctional health care setting. *Journal of Correctional Health Care*, 13(4), pp. 257–267.

Fogarty, L.A., Curbow, B.A., Wingard, J.R., McDonnell, K. and Somerfield, M.R. (1999). Can 40 seconds of compassion reduce patient anxiety? *Journal of Clinical Oncology*, 17(1), pp. 371–379.

Francis, R. (2010). *The Mid Staffordshire NHS Foundation Trust Inquiry. The independent inquiry into care provided by Mid Staffordshire NHS Foundation Trust January 2005–March 2009*. London, UK: The Stationary Office.

Francis, R. (2013). *Report of the Mid Staffordshire NHS Foundation Trust Public Inquiry* (Vol.1–3). London, UK: House of Commons Stationery Office.

Healthcare Commission (2007). *Spotlight on complaints: A report on secod-stage complaints about the NHS in England. Commission for Healthcare Audits and Inspection*. London, UK: Stationery Office.

Hojat, M., Vergare, M.J., Maxwell, K., Brainard, G., Herring, S.K., Isenberg, G.A., Veloski, J. and Gonnella, J.S. (2009). The devil is in the third year: A longitudinal study of erosion of empathy in medical school. *Academic Medicine*, 84(9), pp. 1182–1191.

IBM Corp. (2012). *IBM SPSS statistics for Windows, version 21.0 [computer software]*. New York, NY: Armonk.

Johnson, A. (2008). Speech by the Rt Hon Alan Johnson MP, Secretary of State for Health, 18th June. Manchester, UK: NHS Confederation Annual Conference.

Kret, D. (2011). The qualities of a compassionate nurse according to the perceptions of medical-surgical patients. *Medsurg Nursing*, 20(1), pp. 29–36.

McKenna, H.P. (1994). The Delphi technique: A worthwhile research approach for nursing? Journal of Advanced Nursing, 19(6), pp. 1221–1225.

Mooney, H. (2009). Can you measure compassion? *Nursing Times*. April 2009. Retrieved August 2017 from: www.nursingtimes.net/can-you-measure-compassion/5000543.article.

Neumann, M., Edelhauser, F., Tauschel, D., Fischer, M.R., Wirtz, M., Woopen, C., Haramati, A. and Scheffer, C. (2011). Empathy decline and its reasons: A systematic review of studies with medical students and residents. *Academic Medicine*, 86(8), pp. 996–1009.

Papadopoulos, I. (2011). Courage, compassion and cultural competence. Keynote lecture presented at the 13th Anna Reynvaan Lecture, De Stadsschouwburg – Amsterdam City Theatre. Academic Medical Centre, University of Amsterdam, The Netherlands.

Papadopoulos, I. (2014). The Papadopoulos model for developing culturally competent compassion in healthcare professionals. Retrieved November 2016 from: www.youtube.com/watch?v=zjKzO94TevA.

Papadopoulos, I. and Ali, S. (2015). Measuring compassion in nurses and other healthcare professionals: An integrative review. *Nurse Education in Practice*, 16, pp. 133–139.

Papadopoulos, I., Ali, S. and le Boutillier, N. (in preparation). Development of the Papadopoulos/IENE (Intercultural Education of Nurses in Europe) tool for measuring the nurses' and other healthcare professionals' level of cultural and compassionate competence.

Papadopoulos, I., Tilki, M. and Lees, S. (2004). Promoting cultural competence in health care through a research based intervention in the UK. *Diversity in Health and Social Care*, 1, pp. 107–115.

Petersen, R., Frederiksen, L., Jansen, M.M., Doñate, C., Vidal, C., Castillo, G., …, Ali, S. (2015). Report on integrative literature reviews on: Universal components of compassion. Measuring culturally competent compassion. Learning culturally competent compassion in theory and practice. Intercultural Education of Nurses in Europe (IENE programme) Output 1 of the IENE4 project. Retrieved August 2017 from: http://ieneproject.eu/download/Outputs/Report%20on%20integrative%20%20reviews.pdf.

Qualtrics (2015). *Qualtrics [computer software]*. Provo, UT: Qualtrics.

Roberts, L.W., Warner, T.D., Moutier, C., Geppert, C.M.A. and Hammond, K.A.G. (2011). Are doctors who have been ill more compassionate? Attitudes of resident physicians regarding personal health issues and the expression of compassion in clinical care. *Psychosomatics*, 52, pp. 367–374.

Strauss, C., Taylor, B.L., Gu, J., Kuyken, W., Baer, R., Jones, F., …, Cavanagh, K. (2016). What is compassion and how can we measure it? A review of definitions and measures. *Clinical Psychology Review*, 47, pp. 15–27.

The Patients Association (2009). Patients … not numbers, people … not statistics. Retrieved from: www.patients-association.org.uk/wp-content/uploads/2014/08/Patient-Stories-2009.pdf.

van der Cingel, M. (2011). Compassion in care: A qualitative study of older people with a chronic disease and nurses. *Nursing Ethics*, 18(5), pp. 672–685.

Way, D. and Tracy, S.J. (2012). Conceptualizing compassion as recognizing, relating and (re) acting: A qualitative study of compassionate communication at hospice. *Communication Monographs*, 79(3), pp. 292–315.

10

EPILOGUE

From culturally competent and compassionate humans to culturally competent and compassionate robots

Reflections and conclusions

> Nurses often operate at the margins of human suffering and being exposed to human frailty in ways that few, if any, other occupational groups are, requires that nurses be not only clear about the purpose of nursing practice but also about the need to act in ways that accord with the pursuit of human goods, particularly where achievement of those goods is challenged by the additional vulnerability of being a patient. This requires more than a mere absence of vice…it requires the practice of professional virtue…leading to Aristotle's eudaimonia – translated to mean something akin to 'happiness', 'a good life', 'well-being', or 'flourishing'.
>
> *(Sellman, 2011, p.48)*

I first started planning this book in my head more than five years ago in order to communicate my passion about compassion and my concerns that the nursing profession took compassion for granted and confused (or conflated) the notion of care with that of compassion. I added to these concerns my astonishment regarding the lack of recognition that, although compassion is a universal notion, its understanding and enactment is culturally dependent, something that policy-makers, teachers and researchers had not addressed, resulting in a lack of knowledge and skills in the nursing workforce and health providers in general. My experiences and commitment led me to coin the term 'culturally competent compassion' and soon after to develop my conceptual model of culturally competent compassion. The book I had in mind was going to be my philosophical treatise on culturally competent compassion! But my writing journey took numerous diversions; my original destination was not reached, but naturally evolved into a hybrid of many things: philosophy, practice, politics, policies, proposals, principles, programmes and prescriptions.

In the time that I have taken to complete this book, much has happened, although many would argue little has changed. Incidents of nursing care void of compassion and cultural appropriateness continue to be reported at unacceptable levels, especially in the care of the most vulnerable people. Nursing shortages and a lack of resources are often cited as the root causes of these incidents. In the UK, major changes are on the way in terms of the funding of nursing education, and it is feared that this will result in further reductions in the qualified workforce. The imminent exit of the UK from the European Union most likely will also result in the reduction of the nursing workforce. The changing demography of the country, particularly the growing numbers of the 'very old', demands urgent actions in order to avoid the predictions of distressing and glum consequences unless different and new solutions are found for these challenges.

I found writing this book a challenging journey – challenging because at times I found myself disappointed and sad reading about some of the failures of the profession I love and have devoted all my adult life to. At the same time, the contribution nursing makes to humanity is undisputed. The achievements of many nurses (practitioners, academics, researchers, managers and policy-makers) are impressive. In my journey through the pages of this book, I realised that nursing challenges are healthcare challenges and healthcare challenges are societal and global challenges. Now more than ever, the nursing profession must collaborate with other disciplines and professions for creative solutions. Nursing, with culturally competent compassion at its core, must adapt, adjust, embrace and move ahead in a world dominated by the smart technologies, intelligent computers and social robots able to learn and function autonomously.

Around the same time of my starting this book, I was involved in a HORIZON 2020 application aimed at creating 'socially assistive culturally competent robots' to work in the social care of the elderly. Much of the motivation for this application was the realisation that people are living longer. A recent analysis of global public health data found that people live longer with many more medical problems (Newton, et al., 2015). According to a King's Fund report *Demography: Future trends* (n.d.), in the UK alone, the population of those between sixty-five and eighty-four years of age is projected to increase by 39% by the year 2032, and the number of older adults with healthcare needs is predicted to increase by more than 60%.

Socially assistive robots are sophisticated robots that provide assistance through social interaction using speech, movements, gestures, etc. (Feil-Seifer and Mataric, 2005). Assistive robots can help foster the independence and autonomy of older persons in many ways by reducing the days spent in care institutions and prolonging the time spent living in their own home. Socially assistive robots are currently used in many settings and in healthcare, but attitudes vary over the use of robots, especially in the care of older people.

In our funding application, we argued that if assistive robots are to be accepted in the real world by real people, they must account for the cultural identity and diversity of the assisted person and those of the healthcare team. Following the successful awarding of funding, the CARESSES[1] project was born. Grounded in the work of Papadopoulos (2006) regarding cultural competence, this innovative collaboration of nursing, psychology and robotic and artificial intelligence scientists in a three-year European–Japanese collaborative project aims to create a culturally competent and intelligent robot that can consider both the 'what to do' and the 'how to do' questions.

We have defined a culturally competent robot as a robot that knows general cultural characteristics, but is aware that these general characteristics take different forms in different individuals and can therefore be sensitive to cultural differences while perceiving, reasoning and acting.

The CARESSES team believes that cultural competence will allow assistive robots to increase a user's acceptance of it by being more sensitive to their needs, customs and lifestyle, thus having a greater impact on the quality of life of users and their caregivers, reducing caregiver burden and contributing to the healthcare system's efficiency and effectiveness.

Currently, I have the critical task of developing the guidelines for transcultural robotic nursing, paving the way for future research in this field. The acceptability of robots in healthcare will continue to face challenges, and the continuation of debate among health and social care professionals may lead to the appropriate use of smart technologies amongst different populations and different healthcare problems.

In concluding this book, I feel cautiously optimistic for the future. Although my life's work on cultural competence and culturally competent compassion has been focused on humans (patients, nursing and healthcare students at all levels of education, health and social care organisations and service providers), I believe the time is right to devote some of my time and expertise to a new, inevitable and exciting area of work that deals with artificially intelligent 'beings', which the CARESSES team and I aim to develop so that they will not stereotype and will always be kind and culturally and compassionately competent. I believe that it is important for nurses to be involved and to play a role in the development of future healthcare assistive robotic innovations and to accept the challenge of the increasing need for care with a reduced human workforce in order to ensure that – in the first place – the old and very old people in society continue to receive the culturally competent and compassionate care and support they need. At the same time, culturally competent assistive robots should be used ethically and should be considered as useful tools for human carers, whom they will never replace, but complement.

The legendary broadcaster John Humphrys asked me in an interview on the BBC Radio 4 'Today' programme, "Can we ever have compassionate robots?" My answer was, "We will have a good damn go at it!"

Note

1   CARESSES stands for 'Culturally Aware Robots and Environmental Sensor Systems for Elderly Support'.

References

Feil-Seifer, D. and Mataric, M.J. (2005). Defining socially assistive robots. Proceedings of the 2005 IEEE 9th International Conference on Rehabilitation Robotics, 28 June–1 July 2005, Chicago, IL, pp. 465–468.

King's Fund (n.d.). Demography: Future trends. Retrieved January 2018 from: www.kingsfund.org.uk/projects/time-think-differently/trends-demography

Newton, J.N., Briggs, A.D.M., Murray, C.J.L., Dicker, D., Foreman, K.J., Wang, H., …, Davis, A.C.J. (2015) Changes in health in England, with analysis by English regions and areas of deprivation, 1990–2013: A systematic analysis for the Global Burden of Disease Study 2013. *The Lancet*, 386, pp. 2257–2274.

Papadopoulos, I., ed. (2006). *Transcultural health and social care: Development of culturally competent practitioners*. Edinburgh, UK: Churchill Livingstone Elsevier.

Sellman, D. (2011). *What makes a good nurse*. London, UK: Jessica Kingsley Publishers.

INDEX